The blue zones mediterranean diet cookbook: 250 best kitchen recipes from the healthiest lifestyle on the planet for living longer!

Belinda Turner

Table of Contents

Pistachio Parmesan Kale-Arugula Salad
Pistachio Quinoa Salad with Pomegranate Citrus Vinaigrette
Greek Salad
Creamy Tomato Hummus Soup
Easy Italian Orange and Celery Salad
Cauliflower Tabbouleh Salad
Cucumber Salad
Spicy Sausage Lentil Soup
Spanish Style Turkey Meatball Soup (Instant Pot)
Melon Caprese Salad
Caprese Salad
Vegetable Fagioli
Classic Chicken Broth
Beef Oxtail Soup with White Beans, Tomatoes, and Aleppo Pepper (Instant Pot)
Chopped Greek Antipasto Salad
Roasted Golden Beet, Avocado, and Watercress Salad
Mediterranean Potato Salad
Wild Rice Salad with Chickpeas and Pickled Radish
Chop Chop Salad
Fig and Arugula Salad
Quinoa with Zucchini, Mint, and Pistachios
Panzanella
Summer Panzanella Salad
Sicilian Fish Stew(Instant Pot)
Pastina Chicken soup with kale
Italian White Bean Salad with Bell Peppers
Simple Summer Gazpacho
Watermelon Feta Salad
Roasted Red Pepper Soup with Smoked Paprika and Cilantro Yogurt
Mushroom Barley Soup
French Lentil Salad with Parsley and Mint
Butternut Squash Soup
Easy Pasta Fagioli Soup
Roasted Cauliflower and Arugula Salad with Pomegranate and Pine Nuts
White Bean Soup with Kale
Citrus Fennel Salad
Roasted Carrot Soup with Parmesan Croutons
Red Gazpacho
Lentil Soup
Avgolemono (Lemon Chicken Soup)
Paella Soup
Roasted Eggplant Soup
Chicken and Vegetable Soup

Lentil Sweet Potato Soup
Zucchini and Meatball Soup
Turmeric Red Lentil Soup
Tuscan Bean Soup with Kale
All-Purpose Chicken Broth (Instant Pot)
Moroccan-Style Chickpea Soup
Vegetarian Mains
Socca Pan Pizza with Herbed Ricotta, Fresh Tomato, and Balsamic Glaze
Beet and Watercress Salad with Orange and Dill (Instant Pot)
Cauliflower Steaks with Olive Citrus Sauce
Easy Brussels Sprouts Hash
Caprese-Stuffed Portobellos
Meze Plate with Hummus, Spiced Carrots, and Arugula(Instant Pot)
Walnut Pesto Zoodles
Pistachio Mint Pesto Pasta
Roasted Asparagus with Lemon and Pine Nuts
Mushroom-Leek Tortilla de Patatas
Rustic Garlic Toasts with Stewed Tomatoes, Shaved Fennel, and Burrata (Instnt Pot)
Cauliflower Steaks with Eggplant Relish
Burst Cherry Tomato Sauce with Angel Hair Pasta
Citrus Sautéed Spinach
Gnocchi with Creamy Butternut Squash and Blue Cheese Sauce
Mediterranean Lentil Sloppy Joes
Baked Tofu with Sun-Dried Tomatoes and Artichokes
Mashed Cauliflower
Roasted Ratatouille Pasta
Gorgonzola Sweet Potato Burgers
Baked Mediterranean Tempeh with Tomatoes and Garlic
Broccoli with Ginger and Garlic
Mushroom Ragù with Parmesan Polenta
Garlicky Kale and Parsnips with Soft-Cooked Eggs and Pickled Onions (Instant Pot)
Zucchini-Eggplant Gratin
Roasted Portobello Mushrooms with Kale and Red Onion
Balsamic Roasted Carrots
Braised Fennel with Radicchio, Rear, and Pecorino (Instant Pot)
Grilled Stuffed Portobello Mushrooms
Balsamic Marinated Tofu with Basil and Oregano
Parmesan Zucchini Sticks
Moroccan-Inspired Chickpea Tagine
Green beans with Potatoes and Basil (Instant Pot)
Stuffed Tomatoes with Tabbouleh
Ricotta, Basil, and Pistachio–Stuffed Zucchini
Lemon Kale with Slivered Almonds

5

Pan-Seared Scallops with Sautéed Spinach
Salmon with Wild Rice and Orange Salad (Instant Pot)
Crispy Polenta Fish Sticks
Flounder with Tomatoes and Basil
Pan-Roasted Salmon with Gremolata
Seared Scallops with White Bean Purée
Grilled Mahi-Mahi with Artichoke Caponata
Salmon Burgers
Lemon Pesto Salmon
Hake in Saffron Broth (Instant Pot)
Tuscan Tuna and Zucchini Burgers
Cod and Cauliflower Chowder
Crab Cakes with Shaved Fennel Salad
Shrimp with Arugula Pesto and Zucchini Noodles
Braised Striped Bass with Zucchini and Tomatoes (Instant Pot)
Sardine Bruschetta with Fennel and Lemon Crema
Swordfish Kebabs
Salmon Cakes with Tzatziki Sauce
Halibut with Carrots, White Beans, and Chermoula (Instant Pot)
Mediterranean Cod Stew
Chopped Tuna Salad
Cioppino
Swordfish with Peppers and Potatoes (Instant Pot)
Steamed Mussels in White Wine Sauce
Monkfish with Sautéed Leeks, Fennel, and Tomatoes
Halibut en Papillote with Capers, Onions, Olives, and Tomatoes
Roasted Branzino with Lemon and Herbs
Poultry Mains
Chicken Cutlets with Greek Salsa
Sautéed Chicken Cutlets with Romesco Sauce
Za'atar Rubbed Chicken with Celery Root and Spinach (Instant Pot)
Grilled Oregano Chicken Kebabs with Zucchini and Olives
Crispy Mediterranean Chicken Thighs
Pollock with Roasted Tomatoes
Greek Yogurt–Marinated Chicken Breasts
Honey Almond–Crusted Chicken Tenders
Greek Turkey Burger
Turkey Burgers with Mango Salsa
Bruschetta Chicken Burgers
Chicken and Spiced Freekeh with Cilantro and Preserved Lemon (Instant Pot)
One-Pan Parsley Chicken and Potatoes
Harissa Yogurt Chicken Thighs
Herb-Roasted Turkey Breast

Chicken Gyros with Grilled Vegetables and Tzatziki Sauce
Braised Chicken with Mushrooms and Tomatoes (Instant Pot)
Sumac Chicken with Cauliflower and Carrots
Chicken Sausage and Peppers
Skillet Greek Turkey and Rice
Chicken Tagine (Instant Pot)
Lemon Chicken with Artichokes and Crispy Kale
Chicken Piccata
Lemon and Paprika Herb-Marinated Chicken
Tahini Chicken Rice Bowls
Za'atar Chicken Tenders
One-Pan Tuscan Chicken
Skillet Creamy Tarragon Chicken and Mushrooms
Chicken with Lentils and Butternut Squash (Instant Pot)
Sheet Pan Lemon Chicken and Roasted Artichokes
Chicken Stew with Artichokes, Capers, and Olives
Beef, Pork and Lamb
Spicy Lamb Burgers with Harissa Mayo
Kibbeh
Braised Short Ribs with Fennel and Pickled Grapes
Moroccan Meatballs
Beef Kofta
Dijon and Herb Pork Tenderloin
Wine-Braised Short Ribs with Potatoes (Instant Pot)
Beef Spanakopita Pita Pockets
Mediterranean Chimichurri Skirt Steak
Steak With Red Wine–Mushroom Sauce
Greek-Style Ground Beef Pita Sandwiches
Grilled Steak, Mushroom, and Onion Kebabs
Lamb Meatballs
Greek Meatballs
Lemon Herb-Crusted Pork Tenderloin
Grilled Flank Steak With Grilled Vegetables And Salsa Verde
Italian Salsa Verde
Beef Gyros with Tahini Sauce
Ground Lamb with Lentils and Pomegranate Seeds
Rice and beans
Spiced Rice Pilaf with Sweet Potatoes and Pomegranate (Instant Pot)
Italian Baked Beans
Farro with Artichoke Hearts
Cannellini Bean Lettuce Wraps
Rice and Spinach
Spiced Couscous

7

Table of Contents

Pistachio Parmesan Kale-Arugula Salad
Pistachio Quinoa Salad with Pomegranate Citrus Vinaigrette
Greek Salad
Creamy Tomato Hummus Soup
Easy Italian Orange and Celery Salad
Cauliflower Tabbouleh Salad
Cucumber Salad
Spicy Sausage Lentil Soup
Spanish Style Turkey Meatball Soup (Instant Pot)
Melon Caprese Salad
Caprese Salad
Vegetable Fagioli
Classic Chicken Broth
Beef Oxtail Soup with White Beans, Tomatoes, and Aleppo Pepper (Instant Pot)
Chopped Greek Antipasto Salad
Roasted Golden Beet, Avocado, and Watercress Salad
Mediterranean Potato Salad
Wild Rice Salad with Chickpeas and Pickled Radish
Chop Chop Salad
Fig and Arugula Salad
Quinoa with Zucchini, Mint, and Pistachios
Panzanella
Summer Panzanella Salad
Sicilian Fish Stew(Instant Pot)
Pastina Chicken soup with kale
Italian White Bean Salad with Bell Peppers
Simple Summer Gazpacho
Watermelon Feta Salad
Roasted Red Pepper Soup with Smoked Paprika and Cilantro Yogurt
Mushroom Barley Soup
French Lentil Salad with Parsley and Mint
Butternut Squash Soup
Easy Pasta Fagioli Soup
Roasted Cauliflower and Arugula Salad with Pomegranate and Pine Nuts
White Bean Soup with Kale
Citrus Fennel Salad
Roasted Carrot Soup with Parmesan Croutons
Red Gazpacho
Lentil Soup
Avgolemono (Lemon Chicken Soup)
Paella Soup
Roasted Eggplant Soup
Chicken and Vegetable Soup

Lentil Sweet Potato Soup
Zucchini and Meatball Soup
Turmeric Red Lentil Soup
Tuscan Bean Soup with Kale
All-Purpose Chicken Broth (Instant Pot)
Moroccan-Style Chickpea Soup

Vegetarian Mains

Socca Pan Pizza with Herbed Ricotta, Fresh Tomato, and Balsamic Glaze
Beet and Watercress Salad with Orange and Dill (Instant Pot)
Cauliflower Steaks with Olive Citrus Sauce
Easy Brussels Sprouts Hash
Caprese-Stuffed Portobellos
Meze Plate with Hummus, Spiced Carrots, and Arugula(Instant Pot)
Walnut Pesto Zoodles
Pistachio Mint Pesto Pasta
Roasted Asparagus with Lemon and Pine Nuts
Mushroom-Leek Tortilla de Patatas
Rustic Garlic Toasts with Stewed Tomatoes, Shaved Fennel, and Burrata (Instnt Pot)
Cauliflower Steaks with Eggplant Relish
Burst Cherry Tomato Sauce with Angel Hair Pasta
Citrus Sautéed Spinach
Gnocchi with Creamy Butternut Squash and Blue Cheese Sauce
Mediterranean Lentil Sloppy Joes
Baked Tofu with Sun-Dried Tomatoes and Artichokes
Mashed Cauliflower
Roasted Ratatouille Pasta
Gorgonzola Sweet Potato Burgers
Baked Mediterranean Tempeh with Tomatoes and Garlic
Broccoli with Ginger and Garlic
Mushroom Ragù with Parmesan Polenta
Garlicky Kale and Parsnips with Soft-Cooked Eggs and Pickled Onions (Instant Pot)
Zucchini-Eggplant Gratin
Roasted Portobello Mushrooms with Kale and Red Onion
Balsamic Roasted Carrots
Braised Fennel with Radicchio, Rear, and Pecorino (Instant Pot)
Grilled Stuffed Portobello Mushrooms
Balsamic Marinated Tofu with Basil and Oregano
Parmesan Zucchini Sticks
Moroccan-Inspired Chickpea Tagine
Green beans with Potatoes and Basil (Instant Pot)
Stuffed Tomatoes with Tabbouleh
Ricotta, Basil, and Pistachio–Stuffed Zucchini
Lemon Kale with Slivered Almonds

Sautéed Cabbage with Parsley and Lemon
Braised Radishes with Sugar Snap Peas and Dukkah (Instant Pot)
Farro with Roasted Tomatoes and Mushrooms
Roasted Fennel with Tomatoes
One-Pan Mushroom Pasta with Mascarpone
Spiced Winter Squash with Halloumi and Shaved Brussels Sprouts
North African Peanut Stew Over Cauliflower Rice
Baked Orzo with Eggplant, Swiss Chard, and Mozzarella
Grilled Zucchini with Yogurt and Pomegranate
Lentil Bolognese
Barley Risotto with Tomatoes
Tourli Greek Baked Vegetables
Orzo-Stuffed Tomatoes
Ratatouille
Chickpeas and Kale with Spicy Pomodoro Sauce
Grilled Eggplant Stacks
Roasted Feta with Kale and Lemon Yogurt
Stuffed Red Bell Peppers
Asparagus and Mushroom Farrotto
Roasted Eggplant and Chickpeas with Tomato Sauce
Baked Stuffed Portobello Mushrooms
Sheet Pan Roasted Chickpeas and Vegetables with Harissa Yogurt
Baked Falafel Sliders
Falafel Patties
Quinoa Lentil "Meatballs" With Quick Tomato Sauce
Broiled Eggplant with Basil
Three-Bean Vegetable Chili
Spaghetti Squash Marinara
Braised Fennel with Radicchio and Parmesan
Zucchini Noodles with Peas and Mint

Fish and Seafood Mains

Pistachio-Crusted Whitefish
Poached Salmon (Instant Pot)
Citrus-Glazed Salmon with Zucchini Noodles
Shrimp Scampi
Salmon with Lemon-Garlic Mashed Cauliflower (Instant Pot)
Grilled Fish on Lemons
Salmon Cakes with Bell Pepper and Lemon Yogurt
Shrimp Mojo de Ajo
Easy Shrimp Paella
Salmon with Garlicky Broccoli Rabe and White Beans (Instant Pot)
Weeknight Sheet Pan Fish Dinner
Halibut in Parchment with Zucchini, Shallots, and Herbs

Pan-Seared Scallops with Sautéed Spinach
Salmon with Wild Rice and Orange Salad (Instant Pot)
Crispy Polenta Fish Sticks
Flounder with Tomatoes and Basil
Pan-Roasted Salmon with Gremolata
Seared Scallops with White Bean Purée
Grilled Mahi-Mahi with Artichoke Caponata
Salmon Burgers
Lemon Pesto Salmon
Hake in Saffron Broth (Instant Pot)
Tuscan Tuna and Zucchini Burgers
Cod and Cauliflower Chowder
Crab Cakes with Shaved Fennel Salad
Shrimp with Arugula Pesto and Zucchini Noodles
Braised Striped Bass with Zucchini and Tomatoes (Instant Pot)
Sardine Bruschetta with Fennel and Lemon Crema
Swordfish Kebabs
Salmon Cakes with Tzatziki Sauce
Halibut with Carrots, White Beans, and Chermoula (Instant Pot)
Mediterranean Cod Stew
Chopped Tuna Salad
Cioppino
Swordfish with Peppers and Potatoes (Instant Pot)
Steamed Mussels in White Wine Sauce
Monkfish with Sautéed Leeks, Fennel, and Tomatoes
Halibut en Papillote with Capers, Onions, Olives, and Tomatoes
Roasted Branzino with Lemon and Herbs

Poultry Mains

Chicken Cutlets with Greek Salsa
Sautéed Chicken Cutlets with Romesco Sauce
Za'atar Rubbed Chicken with Celery Root and Spinach (Instant Pot)
Grilled Oregano Chicken Kebabs with Zucchini and Olives
Crispy Mediterranean Chicken Thighs
Pollock with Roasted Tomatoes
Greek Yogurt–Marinated Chicken Breasts
Honey Almond–Crusted Chicken Tenders
Greek Turkey Burger
Turkey Burgers with Mango Salsa
Bruschetta Chicken Burgers
Chicken and Spiced Freekeh with Cilantro and Preserved Lemon (Instant Pot)
One-Pan Parsley Chicken and Potatoes
Harissa Yogurt Chicken Thighs
Herb-Roasted Turkey Breast

Chicken Gyros with Grilled Vegetables and Tzatziki Sauce
Braised Chicken with Mushrooms and Tomatoes (Instant Pot)
Sumac Chicken with Cauliflower and Carrots
Chicken Sausage and Peppers
Skillet Greek Turkey and Rice
Chicken Tagine (Instant Pot)
Lemon Chicken with Artichokes and Crispy Kale
Chicken Piccata
Lemon and Paprika Herb-Marinated Chicken
Tahini Chicken Rice Bowls
Za'atar Chicken Tenders
One-Pan Tuscan Chicken
Skillet Creamy Tarragon Chicken and Mushrooms
Chicken with Lentils and Butternut Squash (Instant Pot)
Sheet Pan Lemon Chicken and Roasted Artichokes
Chicken Stew with Artichokes, Capers, and Olives

Beef, Pork and Lamb

Spicy Lamb Burgers with Harissa Mayo
Kibbeh
Braised Short Ribs with Fennel and Pickled Grapes
Moroccan Meatballs
Beef Kofta
Dijon and Herb Pork Tenderloin
Wine-Braised Short Ribs with Potatoes (Instant Pot)
Beef Spanakopita Pita Pockets
Mediterranean Chimichurri Skirt Steak
Steak With Red Wine–Mushroom Sauce
Greek-Style Ground Beef Pita Sandwiches
Grilled Steak, Mushroom, and Onion Kebabs
Lamb Meatballs
Greek Meatballs
Lemon Herb-Crusted Pork Tenderloin
Grilled Flank Steak With Grilled Vegetables And Salsa Verde
Italian Salsa Verde
Beef Gyros with Tahini Sauce
Ground Lamb with Lentils and Pomegranate Seeds

Rice and beans

Spiced Rice Pilaf with Sweet Potatoes and Pomegranate (Instant Pot)
Italian Baked Beans
Farro with Artichoke Hearts
Cannellini Bean Lettuce Wraps
Rice and Spinach
Spiced Couscous

Bulgur with Chickpeas, Spinach, and Za'atar (Instant Pot)
Mediterranean Lentils and Rice
Sweet Potato Mash
No-Stir Polenta with Arugula, Figs, and Blue Cheese (Instant Pot)
Brown Rice Pilaf with Golden Raisins
Tabbouleh
Brown Rice with Tomatoes and Chickpeas
Wild Mushroom Farrotto (Instant Pot)
Lebanese Rice and Broken Noodles with Cabbage
Orzo with Spinach and Feta
Rice Salad with Oranges, Olives, and Almonds
Barley Salad with Lemon-Tahini Dressing (Instant Pot)
Lemon Farro Bowl with Avocado
Cannellini Bean Salad (Instant Pot)
Barley Risotto with Parmesan
French Lentils with Swiss Chard (Instant pot)
Garlic-Asparagus Israeli Couscous

Simple Sides

Lemon-Thyme Roasted Mixed Vegetables
Roasted Tomato Pita Pizzas
Pasta Puttanesca
Crispy Roasted Red Potatoes with Garlic, Rosemary, and Parmesan
Pasta with Pesto
Spicy Wilted Greens with Garlic
Penne and Fresh Tomato Sauce with Fennel and Orange
Penne and Fresh Tomato Sauce with Spinach and Feta
Couscous with Chicken, Fennel, and Peppers (Instant Pot)
White Clam Pizza Pie
Sun-Dried Tomato and Artichoke Pizza
Roasted Broccolini with Garlic and Romano
Toasted Orzo with Shrimp and Feta
Mediterranean Veggie Pizza with Pourable Thin Crust
Pizza with Arugula and Balsamic Glaze
Roasted Brussels Sprouts with Delicata Squash and Balsamic Glaze
Triple-Green Pasta
Pizza with Red Bell Peppers, Basil, Arugula, and Caramelized Onion
Coriander-Cumin Roasted Carrots
No-Drain Pasta Alla Norma
Flatbread with Olive Tapenade
Garlic and Herb Roasted Grape Tomatoes
Zucchini With Bow Ties
Roasted Cauliflower With Lemon Tahini Sauce
Roasted Asparagus Caprese Pasta

INTRODUCTION

The Blue Zones Mediterranean Diet Cookbook: Kitchen Recipes from the Healthiest Lifestyle on the Planet for Living Longer!

The Blue Zones Mediterranean Diet is known for its health and longevity benefits and the vibrant flavors found in regional staples like sun-ripened tomatoes, savory olive oil, fresh fish, and hearty whole-grain bread.

Whether you're new to this way of life or you grew up eating a Blue Zones Mediterranean Diet, The Blue Zones Mediterranean Diet Cookbook offers flavorful, heart-healthy dishes for everyone.

Bring the Mediterranean Diet--from Italy and Greece to Morocco and Egypt, to Turkey and Lebanon--into your kitchen with more than 100 fresh, flavorful recipes. This comprehensive Blue Zones Mediterranean Diet Cookbook translates the famously healthy Blue Zones Mediterranean Diet for home cooks with a wide range of creative recipes; many are fast enough to be made on a weeknight, using ingredients available at your local supermarket.

The Blue Zones Mediterranean Diet isn't just a way of eating, it's a lifestyle—a complete approach to feeling your best both physically and mentally. The Blue Zones Mediterranean Diet Cookbook makes it easy for you to start and stay on the diet for long-term health.

Changing to a Blue Zones Mediterranean Diet is one of the most important decisions you can make to improve your health, boost energy levels, and also prevent chronic diseases.

People who follow the Blue Zones Mediterranean Diet have a longer life expectancy and lower rates of chronic diseases than do other adults.

And now you have a good chance to get The Blue Zones Mediterranean Diet Cookbook that can help you to save your time and cook super healthy meals.

Please find out how easy it can be to eat well while avoiding food waste. The Blue Zones Mediterranean Diet Cookbook provides you with simple, wellness-boosting recipes that won't leave mountains of leftovers in the fridge.

Discover how this naturally healthy (and delicious) diet can help with heart health, weight management, and more. Dig into a variety of tasty options for everything from breakfast to dessert—all suited for two.

The Blue Zones Mediterranean Diet Cookbook gives you the opportunity to nourish yourself in a simple, affordable, and delicious way.

The Mediterranean Sea is surrounded by an extraordinarily diverse group of countries: Italy, France, and Spain to the north, Greece, Turkey, Israel, Lebanon, and Syria to the east, and to the south, the North African countries of Egypt, Tunisia, Morocco, Algeria, and Libya. This means that there isn't a single "diet" that encompasses the entire Mediterranean region—the spice-laden dishes of Morocco bear little resemblance to the lemon- and caper-laced cuisine of southern Italy. Rather, the Mediterranean diet is about what these cuisines have in common: a daily emphasis on vegetables and fruits, beans and lentils, whole grains, more seafood than meat and poultry, and heart-healthy olive oil. This is the essence of the Mediterranean way of eating and was our overriding principle when deciding what to include in this book.

Changing to a Mediterranean diet is one of the most important decisions you can make to improve your health, boost your energy levels, and also prevent chronic diseases. Science shows that eating more healthily helps you to live longer, it can also help the environment and to reduce the risk of getting sick.

The Mediterranean diet is a very simple style of eating and cooking. It doesn't involve a ton of rules, and it never sacrifices taste or nutrients. Features simple recipes, often rich in beans, vegetables, lean protein, whole grains, herbs, and spices.

My family and I have always loved to cook and experiment in the kitchen, and over the years we've moved more toward the Mediterranean diet. It's partly because of the research on its health benefits, which include lower rates of heart disease, diabetes, cancer, and depression. We also like our food to taste great too, and that's the main reason we've gone Mediterranean.

To help you start thinking about putting the Mediterranean diet into practice, we've compiled a list of recipes that we think work well together.

This book is also beneficial for those people who have wondered about the Mediterranean diet but had absolutely no idea where to start. This Mediterranean diet cookbook is looking forward to help people make changes in their life, starting with their diet.

If you want to start a Mediterranean diet but don't know exactly where to start, don't worry! This book is just for you. Here you can find everything so you can make this change easy and also enjoy it. Here you can find the answers to your questions, advice, and some techniques that you may need.

This cookbook gives you the opportunity to nourish yourself in a simple, affordable, and delicious way. Start cooking with these Mediterranean recipes today as making this change could save your life!

With this cookbook, you will enjoy simple and delicious Mediterranean diet meals that you will love and eat again!

Start cooking with the Blue Zones Mediterranean Diet cookbook today as making this change could save your life!

Welcome to the Blue Zones Mediterranean Diet Cookbook lifestyle.

Enjoy!

Breakfa st
Orange Cardamom Buckwheat Pancakes
PREP: 15 MINUTES • COOK TIME: 10 MINUTES • TOTAL: 25 MINUTES• SERVES: 2

Ingredients

½ cup buckwheat flour

½ teaspoon cardamom

½ teaspoon baking powder

¼ teaspoon baking soda

½ cup milk

¼ cup plain Greek yogurt

1 egg

½ teaspoon orange extract

1 tablespoon maple syrup (optional)

Directions

1. Preparing the Ingredients

In a medium bowl, combine the buckwheat flour, cardamom, baking powder, and baking soda. In another bowl, combine the milk, yogurt, egg, orange extract, and maple syrup (if using) and whisk well to combine. Add the wet ingredients to the dry ingredients and stir until the batter is smooth.

2. Cooking

Heat a nonstick skillet or a griddle over high heat. When the pan is hot, reduce the heat to medium.

Pour the batter into the pan to make four 6-inch pancakes. Depending on the size of your pan, you may need to do this in four batches.

Garlicky Kale And Parsnips With Soft-Cooked Eggs And Pickled Onions (Instant Pot)
PREP: 22 MINUTEs • COOK TIME: 3 MINUTES • TOTAL: 45 MINUTES • SERVES: 4

Ingredients

12 ounces parsnips, peeled

2 tablespoons extra-virgin olive oil, plus extra for drizzling

4 garlic cloves, minced

2 pounds kale, stemmed and cut into 1-inch pieces

¾ cup chicken or vegetable broth

½ teaspoon table salt

4 large eggs

¼ cup Quick Pickled Onions

½ cup Lemon-Yogurt Sauce

1 teaspoon ground dried Aleppo pepper

Directions

1. Preparing the Ingredients

Cut parsnips into 2-inch lengths. Leave thin pieces whole, halve medium pieces lengthwise, and quarter thick pieces lengthwise.

2. Cooking

Using highest sauté function, cook oil and garlic in Instant Pot until fragrant, about 1 minute. Stir in half of kale and cook until slightly wilted, about 1 minute. Add remaining kale and repeat. Stir in broth and salt, then add parsnips.

Lock lid in place and close pressure release valve. Select high pressure cook function and cook for 3 minutes.

Turn off Instant Pot and quick-release pressure. Carefully remove lid, allowing steam to escape away from you. Season kale and parsnips with salt and pepper to taste. Transfer to bowl and cover to keep warm. Discard cooking liquid in pot.

Arrange trivet included with Instant Pot in base of now-empty insert and add 1 cup water. Using highest sauté function, bring water to boil. Set eggs on trivet. Lock lid in place and close pressure release valve. Select high pressure cook function and set cook time for 3 minutes. Cook eggs for 2½ minutes (fully set whites with runny yolks) or 3 minutes (fully set whites with fudgy yolks). Turn off Instant Pot and quick-release pressure. Carefully remove lid, allowing steam to escape away from you. Using tongs, transfer eggs to separate bowl and place under cold running water for 30 seconds. Drain and peel eggs. Divide kale and parsnips among individual serving bowls. Top with pickled onions, yogurt sauce, and eggs. Sprinkle with Aleppo pepper and drizzle with extra oil. Serve.

Sunny-Side Up Baked Eggs With Swiss Chard, Feta, And Basil

PREP: 15 MINUTES • COOK TIME: 10 TO 15 MINUTES • TOTAL: 30 MINUTES • SERVES: 4

Ingredients

1 tablespoon extra-virgin olive oil, divided

½ red onion, diced

½ teaspoon kosher salt

¼ teaspoon nutmeg

⅛ teaspoon freshly ground black pepper

4 cups Swiss chard, chopped

¼ cup crumbled feta cheese

4 large eggs

¼ cup fresh basil, chopped or cut into ribbons

Directions

1. Preparing the Ingredients

Preheat the oven to 375°F. Place 4 ramekins on a half sheet pan or in a baking dish and grease lightly with olive oil.

2. Cooking

Heat the remaining olive oil in a large skillet or sauté pan over medium heat. Add the onion, salt, nutmeg, and pepper and sauté until translucent, about 3 minutes. Add the chard and cook, stirring, until wilted, about 2 minutes.

Split the mixture among the 4 ramekins. Add 1 tablespoon feta cheese to each ramekin. Crack 1 egg on top of the mixture in each ramekin. Bake for 10 to 12 minutes, or until the egg white is set.

Allow to cool for 1 to 2 minutes, then carefully transfer the eggs from the ramekins to a plate with a fork or spatula. Garnish with the basil.

Julene's Green Juice

PREP: 5 MINUTES • COOK TIME: NONE • TOTAL: 5 MINUTES• TOTAL: 5 MINUTES • SERVES: 1

Ingredients

3 cups dark leafy greens

1 cucumber

¼ cup fresh Italian parsley leaves

¼ pineapple, cut into wedges

½ green apple

½ orange

½ lemon

Directions

1. Preparing the Ingredients

Pinch grated fresh ginger. Using a juicer, run the greens, cucumber, parsley, pineapple, apple, orange, lemon, and ginger through it, pour into a large cup, and serve.

Strawberry Basil Honey Ricotta Toast

PREP: 10 MINUTES • COOK TIME: 30 MINUTES • TOTAL: 40 MINUTES • SERVES: 2

Ingredients

4 slices of whole-grain bread
½ cup ricotta cheese (whole milk or low-fat)
1 tablespoon honey
Sea salt
1 cup fresh strawberries, sliced
4 large fresh basil leaves, sliced into thin shreds

Directions

1. Preparing the Ingredients.

Toast the bread. In a small bowl, combine the ricotta, honey, and a pinch or two of sea salt. Taste and add additional honey or salt if desired. Spread the mixture evenly over each slice of bread (about 2 tablespoons per slice). Top each piece with sliced strawberries and a few pieces of shredded basil.

Ricotta cheese is often overlooked unless you're making lasagna for a crowd. However, it's a great source of protein and full of calcium. It's also a nice, silky-smooth spreadable cheese that you can make sweet or savory for a meal or snack. Spread it on high-fiber whole-grain toast and top it with fruit. Perfect for a quick breakfast or afternoon snack.

Greek Yogurt Breakfast Parfaits With Roasted Grapes

PREP: 5 MINUTES • COOK TIME: 25 MINUTES • TOTAL: 30 MINUTES• SERVES: 4

Ingredients

1½ pounds seedless grapes (about 4 cups)

1 tablespoon extra-virgin olive oil

2 cups 2% plain Greek yogurt

½ cup chopped walnuts

4 teaspoons honey

Directions

1. Preparing the Ingredients

Place a large, rimmed baking sheet in the oven. Preheat the oven to 450°F with the pan inside.

Wash the grapes and remove from the stems. Dry on a clean kitchen towel, and put in a bowl. Drizzle with the oil, and toss to coat.

2. Cooking .

Carefully remove the hot pan from the oven, and pour the grapes onto the pan. Bake for 20 to 23 minutes, until slightly shriveled, stirring once halfway through. Remove the baking sheet from the oven and cool on a wire rack for 5 minutes.

While the grapes are cooling, assemble the parfaits by spooning the yogurt into four bowls or tall glasses. Top each bowl or glass with 2 tablespoons of walnuts and 1 teaspoon of honey.

When the grapes are slightly cooled, top each parfait with a quarter of the grapes. Scrape any accumulated sweet grape juice onto the parfaits and serve.

Chocolate Banana Smoothie

PREP: 5 MINUTES • COOK TIME: NONE • TOTAL: 5 MINUTES• SERVES: 2

Ingredients

2 bananas, peeled

1 cup unsweetened almond milk, or skim milk

1 cup crushed ice

3 tablespoons unsweetened cocoa powder

3 tablespoons honey

Directions

1. Preparing the Ingredients

Smoothies are great for breakfast on the go because they are quick, fill you up, and provide lasting energy throughout the morning. You can refrigerate leftovers and reblend the next day for about 30 seconds on high speed. In a blender, combine the bananas, almond milk, ice, cocoa powder, and honey. Blend until smooth.

Cherry Almond Baked Oatmeal Cups

PREP: 10 MINUTES, PLUS 10 MINUTES TO COOL • COOK TIME: 35-45 MINUTES • TOTAL: 1 HOUR• SERVES: 6

Ingredients

½ cup gluten-free old-fashioned oats

2 tablespoons sliced almonds
Pinch salt
¾ cup milk
½ teaspoon almond extract
½ teaspoon vanilla
1 egg, beaten
2 tablespoons maple syrup
1 cup frozen cherries, thawed
Ricotta cheese (optional, for topping)
Greek yogurt (optional, for topping)

Directions

1. Preparing the Ingredients

Preheat the oven to 350°F and set the rack to the middle position. Oil two 8-ounce ramekins and place them on a baking sheet. In a medium bowl, combine all of the ingredients and mix well. Spoon half of the mixture into each ramekin.

2. Cooking

Bake for 35 to 45 minutes, or until the oats are set and a knife inserted into the middle comes out clean. They will be soft but should not be runny.

Let the baked oats cool for 5 to 10 minutes. Top with ricotta cheese or plain Greek yogurt, if desired.

Mashed Chickpea, Feta, And Avocado Toast

PREP: 10 MINUTES • COOK TIME: 15 MINUTES • TOTAL: 25 MINUTES• SERVES: 4

Ingredients

1 (15-ounce) can chickpeas, drained and rinsed

1 avocado, pitted

½ cup diced feta cheese (about 2 ounces)

2 teaspoons freshly squeezed lemon juice or 1 tablespoon orange juice

½ teaspoon freshly ground black pepper

4 pieces multigrain toast

2 teaspoons honey

Directions

1. Preparing the Ingredients

Put the chickpeas in a large bowl. Scoop the avocado flesh into the bowl.

With a potato masher or large fork, mash the ingredients together until the mix has a spreadable consistency. It doesn't need to be totally smooth. Add the feta, lemon juice, and pepper, and mix well.

Evenly divide the mash onto the four pieces of toast and spread with a knife. Drizzle with honey and serve.

Egg In A "Pepper Hole" With Avocado

PREP: 15 MINUTES • COOK TIME: 5 MINUTES • TOTAL: 20 MINUTES• SERVES: 4

Ingredients

4 bell peppers, any color

1 tablespoon extra-virgin olive oil

8 large eggs

¾ teaspoon kosher salt, divided

¼ teaspoon freshly ground black pepper, divided

1 avocado, peeled, pitted, and diced

¼ cup red onion, diced

¼ cup fresh basil, chopped

Juice of ½ lime

Directions

1. Preparing the Ingredients

Stem and seed the bell peppers. Cut 2 (2-inch-thick) rings from each pepper. Chop the remaining bell pepper into small dice, and set aside.

2. Cooking

Heat the olive oil in a large skillet over medium heat. Add 4 bell pepper rings, then crack 1 egg in the middle of each ring. Season with ¼ teaspoon of the salt and ⅛ teaspoon of the black pepper. Cook until the egg whites are mostly set but the yolks are still runny, 2 to 3 minutes. Gently flip and cook 1 additional minute for over easy. Move the egg–bell pepper rings to a platter or onto plates, and repeat with the remaining 4 bell pepper rings.

In a medium bowl, combine the avocado, onion, basil, lime juice, reserved diced bell pepper, the remaining ¼ teaspoon kosher salt, and the remaining ⅛ teaspoon black pepper. Divide among the 4 plates.

Fruit Smoothie

PREP: 5 MINUTES • COOK TIME: NONE • TOTAL: 5 MINUTES• SERVES: 2

Ingredients

2 cups blueberries (or any fresh or frozen fruit, cut into pieces if the fruit is large)
2 cups unsweetened almond milk
1 cup crushed ice
½ teaspoon ground ginger (or other dried ground spice such as turmeric, cinnamon, or nutmeg)

Directions

1. Preparing the Ingredients

In a blender, combine the blueberries, almond milk, ice, and ginger. Blend until smooth. Some flavor combinations to try: ginger and blueberry, honeydew melon and turmeric, mango and nutmeg, or mixed berries and cinnamon. Have fun experimenting!

The great thing about fruit smoothies is how easy it is to customize them using-seasonal produce. Because fruit is naturally sweet, you don't need to add any additional sweetener here. If using seasonal fruits, opt for fresh. In the absence of seasonal fruits, use frozen fruits.

Individual Baked Egg Casseroles

PREP: 10 MINUTES • COOK TIME: 30 MINUTES • TOTAL: 40 MINUTES• SERVES: 2

Ingredients

1 slice whole-grain bread

4 large eggs, beaten

3 tablespoons milk

¼ teaspoon salt

½ teaspoon onion powder

¼ teaspoon garlic powder

Pinch freshly ground black pepper

¾ cup chopped vegetables (any kind you like)

Directions

1. Preparing the Ingredients

Heat the oven to 375°F and set the rack to the middle position. Oil two 8-ounce ramekins and place them on a baking sheet. Tear the bread into pieces and line each ramekin with ½ of a slice. Mix the eggs, milk, salt, onion powder, garlic powder, pepper, and vegetables in a medium bowl. Pour half of the egg mixture into each ramekin.

2. Cooking

Bake for 30 minutes, or until the eggs are set.

Quickie Honey Nut Granola

PREP: 10 MINUTES • COOK TIME: 20 MINUTES • TOTAL: 30 MINUTES• SERVES: 6

Ingredients

2½ cups regular rolled oats

⅓ cup coarsely chopped almonds

⅛ teaspoon kosher or sea salt

½ teaspoon ground cinnamon

½ cup chopped dried apricots

2 tablespoons ground flaxseed

¼ cup honey

¼ cup extra-virgin olive oil

2 teaspoons vanilla extract

Directions

1. Preparing the Ingredients

Preheat the oven to 325°F. Line a large, rimmed baking sheet with parchment paper.

2. Cooking

n a large skillet, combine the oats, almonds, salt, and cinnamon. Turn the heat to medium-high and cook, stirring often, to toast, about 6 minutes. While the oat mixture is toasting, in a microwave-safe bowl, combine the apricots, flaxseed, honey, and oil. Microwave on high for about 1 minute, or until very hot and just beginning to bubble. (Or heat these ingredients in a small saucepan over medium heat for about 3 minutes.) Stir the vanilla into the honey mixture, then pour it over the oat mixture in the skillet. Stir well.

Spread out the granola on the prepared baking sheet. Bake for 15 minutes, until lightly browned. Remove from the oven and cool completely. Break the granola into small pieces, and store in an airtight container in the refrigerator for up to 2 weeks.

Polenta With Sautéed Chard And Fried Eggs

PREP: 5 MINUTES • COOK TIME: 20 MINUTES • TOTAL: 25 MINUTES• SERVES: 4

Ingredients

2½ cups water

½ teaspoon kosher salt

¾ cups whole-grain cornmeal

¼ teaspoon freshly ground black pepper

2 tablespoons grated Parmesan cheese

1 tablespoon extra-virgin olive oil

1 bunch (about 6 ounces) Swiss chard, leaves and stems chopped and separated

2 garlic cloves, sliced

¼ teaspoon kosher salt

⅛ teaspoon freshly ground black pepper

Lemon juice (optional)

1 tablespoon extra-virgin olive oil

4 large eggs

Directions

1. Preparing the Ingredients

Bring the water and salt to a boil in a medium saucepan over high heat. Slowly add the cornmeal, whisking constantly. Decrease the heat to low, cover, and cook for 10 to 15 minutes, stirring often to avoid lumps. Stir in the pepper and Parmesan, and divide among 4 bowls.

2. Cooking

Heat the oil in a large skillet over medium heat. Add the chard stems, garlic, salt, and pepper; sauté for 2 minutes. Add the chard leaves and cook until wilted, about 3 to 5 minutes. Add a spritz of lemon juice (if desired), toss together, and divide evenly on top of the polenta.

Heat the oil in the same large skillet over medium-high heat. Crack each egg into the skillet, taking care not to crowd the skillet and leaving space between the eggs. Cook until the whites are set and golden around the edges, about 2 to 3 minutes.

Serve sunny-side up or flip the eggs over carefully and cook 1 minute longer for over easy. Place one egg on top of the polenta and chard in each bowl.

Berry And Yogurt Parfait

PREP: 5 MINUTES • COOK TIME: NONE • TOTAL: 5 MINUTES• SERVES: 2

Ingredients

1 cup raspberries

1½ cups unsweetened nonfat plain Greek yogurt

1 cup blackberries

¼ cup chopped walnuts

Directions

Preparing the Ingredients

In 2 bowls, layer the raspberries, yogurt, and blackberries. Sprinkle with the walnuts.

You can use any berries you like here, but the raspberries and blackberries in this recipe add a nice variety of flavors, and they don't require any chopping. These parfaits are especially good in the summer when berries are in season. Feel free to substitute any chopped fresh fruit.

Overnight Pomegranate Muesli

PREP: 10 MINUTES, PLUS OVERNIGHT TO CHILL • COOK TIME: 30 MINUTES • TOTAL: 40 MINUTES• SERVES: 2

Ingredients

½ cup gluten-free old-fashioned oats

¼ cup shelled pistachios

3 tablespoons pumpkin seeds

2 tablespoons chia seeds

¾ cup milk

½ cup plain Greek yogurt

2 to 3 teaspoons maple syrup (optional)

½ cup pomegranate arils

Directions

Preparing the Ingredients

In a medium bowl, mix together the oats, pistachios, pumpkin seeds, chia seeds, milk, yogurt, and maple syrup, if using.

Divide the mixture between two 12-ounce mason jars or another type of container with a lid.

Top each with ¼ cup of pomegranate arils.

Cover each jar or container and store in the refrigerator overnight or up to 4 days.

Serve cold, with additional milk if desired.

Breakfast Polenta

PREP: 5 MINUTES • COOK TIME: 10 MINUTES • TOTAL: 15 MINUTES• SERVES: 6

Ingredients

2 (18-ounce) tubes plain polenta

2¼ to 2½ cups 2% milk, divided

2 oranges, peeled and chopped

½ cup chopped pecans

¼ cup 2% plain Greek yogurt

8 teaspoons honey

Directions

Preparing the Ingredients

1. Slice the polenta into rounds and place in a microwave-safe bowl. Heat in the microwave on high for 45 seconds.

Transfer the polenta to a large pot, and mash it with a potato masher or fork until coarsely mashed. Place the pot on the stove over medium heat.

2. In a medium, microwave-safe bowl, heat the milk in the microwave on high for 1 minute. Pour 2 cups of the warmed milk into the pot with the polenta, and stir with a whisk. Continue to stir and mash with the whisk, adding the remaining

milk a few tablespoons at a time, until the polenta is fairly smooth and heated through, about 5 minutes. Remove from the stove.

3. Divide the polenta among four serving bowls. Top each bowl with one-quarter of the oranges, 2 tablespoons of pecans, 1 tablespoon of yogurt, and 2 teaspoons of honey before serving.

Smoked Salmon Egg Scramble With Dill And Chives

PREP: 5 MINUTES • COOK TIME: 5 MINUTES • TOTAL: 10 MINUTES • SERVES: 2

Ingredients
4 large eggs
1 tablespoon milk
1 tablespoon fresh chives, minced
1 tablespoon fresh dill, minced
¼ teaspoon kosher salt
⅛ teaspoon freshly ground black pepper
2 teaspoons extra-virgin olive oil
2 ounces smoked salmon, thinly sliced

Directions
1. Preparing the Ingredients
In a large bowl, whisk together the eggs, milk, chives, dill, salt, and pepper.

2. Cooking
Heat the olive oil in a medium skillet or sauté pan over medium heat. Add the egg mixture and cook for about 3 minutes, stirring occasionally.

Add the salmon and cook until the eggs are set but moist, about 1 minute.

Yogurt With Blueberries, Honey, And Mint

PREP: 5 MINUTES • COOK TIME: NONE• TOTAL: 5 MINUTES• SERVES: 2

Ingredients
2 cups unsweetened nonfat plain Greek yogurt
1 cup blueberries
3 tablespoons honey
2 tablespoons fresh mint leaves, chopped

Directions
Preparing the Ingredients
Apportion the yogurt between 2 small bowls. Top with the blueberries, honey, and mint.

Mediterranean Breakfast Pizza

PREP: 5 MINUTES • COOK TIME: 15 MINUTES • TOTAL: 20 MINUTES• SERVES: 2

Ingredients
2 (6- to 8-inch-long) pieces of whole-wheat naan bread
2 tablespoons prepared pesto
1 medium tomato, sliced
2 large eggs

Directions

1. Preparing the Ingredients

Heat a large nonstick skillet over medium-high heat. Place the naan bread in the skillet and let it warm for about 2 minutes on each side. The bread should be softened and just starting to turn golden. Spread 1 tablespoon of the pesto on one side of each slice. Top the pesto with tomato slices to cover. Remove the pizzas from the pan and place each one on its own plate.

Crack the eggs into the pan, keeping them separated, and cook until the whites are no longer translucent and the yolk is cooked to desired doneness. With a spatula, spoon one egg onto each pizza.

Snacks and Sides
White Bean Harissa Dip

PREP TIME: 10 MINUTES / COOK TIME: 1 HOUR / TOTAL: 1 HOUR 10 MINUTES / MAKES 1½ CUPS

Ingredients

1 whole head of garlic

½ cup olive oil, divided

1 (15-ounce) can cannellini beans, drained and rinsed

1 teaspoon salt

1 teaspoon harissa paste (or more to taste)

Directions

1. Preparing the Ingredients

Preheat the oven to 350°F.

Cut about ½ inch off the top of a whole head of garlic and lightly wrap it in foil. Drizzle 1 to 2 teaspoons of olive oil over the top of the cut side.

2. Cooking

Place it in an oven-safe dish and roast it in the oven for about 1 hour or until the cloves are soft and tender.

Remove the garlic from the oven and let it cool. The garlic can be roasted up to 2 days ahead of time.

Remove the garlic cloves from their skin and place them in the bowl of a food processor along with the beans, salt, and harissa. Purée, drizzling in as much olive oil as needed until the beans are smooth. If the dip seems too stiff, add additional olive oil to loosen the dip. Taste the dip and add additional salt, harissa, or oil as needed.

Store in the refrigerator for up to a week. Portion out ¼ cup of dip and serve with a mixture of raw vegetables and mini pita breads.

Mediterranean Fruit, Veggie, and Cheese Board

PREP TIME: 15 MINUTES / COOK TIME: 1 HOUR / TOTAL: 1 HOUR PLUS 15 MINUTES / SERVES 4

Ingredients

2 cups sliced fruits, such as apples, pears, plums, or peaches

2 cups finger-food fruits, such as berries, cherries, grapes, or figs

2 cups raw vegetables cut into sticks, such as carrots, celery, broccoli, cauliflower, or whole cherry tomatoes

1 cup cured, canned, or jarred vegetables, such as roasted peppers or artichoke hearts, or ½ cup olives

1 cup cubed cheese, such as goat cheese, Gorgonzola, feta, Manchego, or Asiago (about 4 ounces)

Directions

Preparing the Ingredients

1. Wash all the fresh produce and cut into slices or bite-size pieces, as described in the ingredients list.

2. Arrange all the ingredients on a wooden board or serving tray. Include small spoons for items like the berries and olives, and a fork or knife for the cheeses. Serve with small plates and napkins.

Summer Squash Ribbons with Lemon and Ricotta

PREP TIME: 20 MINUTES / COOK TIME: 1 HOUR / TOTAL: 1 HOUR 20 MINUTES / MAKES ½ CUPS

Ingredients

2 medium zucchini or yellow squash
½ cup ricotta cheese
2 tablespoons fresh mint, chopped, plus additional mint leaves for garnish
2 tablespoons fresh parsley, chopped
Zest of ½ lemon
2 teaspoons lemon juice
½ teaspoon kosher salt
¼ teaspoon freshly ground black pepper
1 tablespoon extra-virgin olive oil

Directions

Preparing the Ingredients

1. Using a vegetable peeler, make ribbons by peeling the summer squash lengthwise.
The squash ribbons will resemble the wide pasta, pappardelle.
2. In a medium bowl, combine the ricotta cheese, mint, parsley, lemon zest, lemon juice, salt, and black pepper. Place mounds of the squash ribbons evenly on 4 plates then dollop the ricotta mixture on top. Drizzle with the olive oil and garnish with the mint leaves.

HUMMUS

PREP TIME: 10 MINUTES / COOK TIME: 30 MINUTES/ TOTAL: 40 MINUTES / MAKES 1-4 OUNCE

Ingredients

1 (14-ounce) can chickpeas, drained
3 garlic cloves, minced
2 tablespoons tahini
2 tablespoons extra-virgin olive oil
Juice of 1 lemon
Zest of 1 lemon
½ teaspoon sea salt
Pinch cayenne pepper
2 tablespoons chopped fresh Italian parsley leaves

Directions

Preparing the Ingredients

1. In a blender, combine the chickpeas, garlic, tahini, olive oil, lemon juice and zest, sea salt and cayenne. Blend for about 60 seconds until smooth. Garnish with parsley and serve.

Mediterranean Trail Mix

PREP TIME: 10 MINUTES / COOK TIME: 10 MINUTES/ TOTAL: 20 MINUTES / MAKES 4 CUPS

Ingredients

1 tablespoon olive oil

1 tablespoon maple syrup

1 teaspoon vanilla

½ teaspoon cardamom

½ teaspoon allspice

2 cups mixed, unsalted nuts

¼ cup unsalted pumpkin or sunflower seeds

½ cup dried apricots, diced or thin sliced

½ cup dried figs, diced or thinly sliced

Pinch salt

Directions

1. **Preparing the Ingredients.** Combine the olive oil, maple syrup, vanilla, cardamom, and allspice in a large sauté pan over medium heat. Stir to combine. Add the nuts and seeds and stir well to coat. Let the nuts and seeds toast for about 10 minutes, stirring frequently. Remove from the heat, and add the dried apricots and figs. Stir everything well and season with salt. Store in an airtight container. Nuts are a great thing to buy in bulk. As long as you store them in airtight containers, they'll last for a few months. Look for raw nuts that don't have added salt or sugar. That way you can toast them and flavor them in any way you like.

Quick Toasted Almonds

PREP TIME: 10 MINUTES / COOK TIME: 30 MINUTES/ MAKES 2 CUPS

Ingredients

1 tablespoon extra-virgin olive oil

2 cups skin-on raw whole almonds

1 teaspoon salt

¼ teaspoon pepper

Directions

1. **Preparing the Ingredients**

Heat oil in 12-inch nonstick skillet over medium-high heat until just shimmering. Add almonds, salt, and pepper and reduce heat to medium-low. Cook, stirring often, until almonds are fragrant and their color deepens slightly, about 8 minutes. Transfer almonds to paper towel–lined plate and let cool before serving. (Almonds can be stored at room temperature for up to 5 days.)

Lemony Garlic Hummus

PREP TIME: 10 MINUTES / COOK TIME: NONE / SERVES 6

Ingredients

1 (15-ounce) can chickpeas

Drained

Liquid reserved

3 tablespoons freshly squeezed lemon juice (from about 1 large lemon)

2 tablespoons peanut butter

3 tablespoons extra-virgin olive oil, divided

2 garlic cloves

¼ teaspoon kosher or sea salt (optional)

Raw veggies or whole-grain crackers, for serving (optional)

Directions

1. Preparing the Ingredients

In the bowl of a food processor, combine the chickpeas and 2 tablespoons of the reserved chickpea liquid with the lemon juice, peanut butter, 2 tablespoons of oil, and the garlic. Process the mixture for 1 minute. Scrape down the sides of the bowl with a rubber spatula. Process for 1 more minute, or until smooth.

Put in a serving bowl, drizzle with the remaining 1 tablespoon of olive oil, sprinkle with the salt, if using, and serve with veggies or crackers, if desired.

The key to light, airy hummus is to add some chickpea liquid, also known as aquafaba. While we usually recommend draining and rinsing canned beans to remove more sodium, for this recipe, save that liquid gold to make your hummus beyond delicious.

Sautéed Kale with Tomato and Garlic

PREP TIME: 10 MINUTES / COOK TIME: 5 MINUTES/ MAKES 14.5 OUNCE/ SERVES 4

Ingredients

1 tablespoon extra-virgin olive oil

4 garlic cloves, sliced

¼ teaspoon red pepper flakes

2 bunches kale, stemmed and chopped or torn into pieces

1 (14.5-ounce) can no-salt-added diced tomatoes

½ teaspoon kosher salt

Directions

1. Preparing the Ingredients

Heat the olive oil in a wok or large skillet over medium-high heat. Add the garlic and red pepper flakes, and sauté until fragrant, about 30 seconds. Add the kale and sauté, about 3 to 5 minutes, until the kale shrinks down a bit. Add the tomatoes and the salt, stir together, and cook for 3 to 5 minutes, or until the liquid reduces and the kale cooks down further and becomes tender. Adding garlic and red pepper flakes to the oil first allows the flavors to permeate the oil, creating more flavor for the overall dish. If this makes the dish too spicy for your palate, eliminate the red pepper flakes or add them in step 2 with the salt and tomatoes.

Baba Ganoush

PREP TIME: 10 MINUTES / COOK TIME: 15 MINUTES/ MAKES ½ CUP

Ingredients

1 eggplant, peeled and sliced
¼ cup tahini
½ teaspoon sea salt
Juice of 1 lemon
¼ teaspoon ground cumin
⅛ teaspoon freshly ground black pepper
2 tablespoons extra-virgin olive oil
2 tablespoons sunflower seeds (optional)
2 tablespoons fresh Italian parsley leaves (optional)

Directions

1. Preparing the Ingredients

Preheat the oven to 350°F. On a baking sheet, spread the eggplant slices in an even layer.

2. Cooking

Bake for about 15 minutes until soft. Cool slightly and roughly chop the eggplant. In a blender, blend the eggplant with the tahini, sea salt, lemon juice, cumin, and pepper for about 30 seconds. Transfer to a serving dish. Drizzle with the olive oil and sprinkle with the sunflower seeds and parsley (if using) before serving. You can also make Baba Ganoush with zucchini in place of the eggplant. Halve 4 zucchini lengthwise (no need to peel!) and cook in a 350°F oven for about 10 minutes until soft. Continue with the recipe as directed.

Seared Halloumi with Pesto and Tomato

PREP TIME: 2 MINUTES / COOK TIME: 5 MINUTES/ MAKES ½ CUPS

Ingredients

3 ounces Halloumi cheese, cut crosswise into 2 thinner, rectangular pieces

2 teaspoons prepared pesto sauce, plus additional for drizzling if desired

1 medium tomato, sliced

Directions

1. Preparing the Ingredients

Heat a nonstick skillet over medium-high heat and place the slices of Halloumi in the hot pan. After about 2 minutes, check to see if the cheese is golden on the bottom. If it is, flip the slices, top each with 1 teaspoon of pesto, and cook for another 2 minutes, or until the second side is golden. Serve with slices of tomato and a drizzle of pesto, if desired, on the side. Because Halloumi is a fairly salty cheese, no additional salt is needed in this dish.

Romesco Dip

PREP TIME: 10 MINUTES / COOK TIME: NONE/ MAKES 12 OUNCE / SERVES 10

Ingredients

1 (12-ounce) jar roasted red peppers, drained

1 (14.5-ounce) can diced tomatoes, undrained

½ cup dry-roasted almonds

2 garlic cloves

2 teaspoons red wine vinegar

1 teaspoon smoked paprika or ½ teaspoon cayenne pepper

¼ teaspoon kosher or sea salt

¼ teaspoon freshly ground black pepper

¼ cup extra-virgin olive oil

⅔ cup torn, day-old bread or toast (about 2 slices)

Assortment of sliced raw vegetables such as carrots, celery, cucumber, green beans, and bell peppers, for serving

Directions

1. Preparing the Ingredients

In a high-powered blender or food processor, combine the roasted peppers, tomatoes and their juices, almonds, garlic, vinegar, smoked paprika, salt, and pepper. Begin puréeing the ingredients on medium speed, and slowly drizzle in the oil with the blender running. Continue to purée until the dip is thoroughly mixed. Add the bread and purée.

Serve with raw vegetables for dipping, or store in a jar with a lid for up to one week in the refrigerator.

Roasted Broccoli with Tahini Yogurt Sauce

PREP TIME: 15 MINUTES / COOK TIME: 30 MINUTES/ MAKES ½ CUPS / SERVES 4

Ingredients

1½ to 2 pounds broccoli, stalk trimmed and cut into slices, head cut into florets
1 lemon, sliced into ¼-inch-thick rounds
3 tablespoons extra-virgin olive oil
½ teaspoon kosher salt
¼ teaspoon freshly ground black pepper
½ cup plain Greek yogurt
2 tablespoons tahini
1 tablespoon lemon juice
¼ teaspoon kosher salt
1 teaspoon sesame seeds, for garnish (optional)

Directions

1. Preparing the Ingredients

Preheat the oven to 425°F. Line a baking sheet with parchment paper or foil.
In a large bowl, gently toss the broccoli, lemon slices, olive oil, salt, and black pepper to combine. Arrange the broccoli in a single layer on the prepared baking sheet.

2. Cooking

Roast 15 minutes, stir, and roast another 15 minutes, until golden brown. In a medium bowl, combine the yogurt, tahini, lemon juice, and salt; mix well. Spread the tahini yogurt sauce on a platter or large plate and top with the broccoli and lemon slices. Garnish with the sesame seeds (if desired). Lining your baking sheet with parchment paper or foil makes cleanup a breeze. Simply crumple up and throw away with no need to scrub brown bits off the pan.

Spiced Almonds

PREP TIME: 10 MINUTES / COOK TIME: 7 MINUTES/ MAKES ½ CUPS / SERVES 8

Ingredients

2 cups raw unsalted almonds

1 tablespoon extra-virgin olive oil

1 teaspoon ground cumin

½ teaspoon garlic powder

½ teaspoon sea salt

⅛ teaspoon cayenne pepper

Directions

1. Preparing the Ingredients

In a large nonstick skillet over medium-high heat, cook the almonds for about 3 minutes, shaking the pan constantly, until the almonds become fragrant. Transfer to a bowl and set aside. In the same skillet over medium-high heat, heat the olive oil until it shimmers. Add the cumin, garlic powder, sea salt, and cayenne. Cook for 30 to 60 seconds, until the spices become fragrant. Add the almonds to the skillet. Cook for about 3 minutes more, stirring, until the spices coat the almonds. Let cool before serving.

Stuffed Cucumber Cups

PREP TIME: 5 MINUTES / COOK TIME: 30 MINUTES/ MAKES 8 OUNCES / SERVES 2

Ingredients

1 medium cucumber (about 8 ounces, 8 to 9 inches long)

½ cup hummus (any flavor) or white bean dip

4 or 5 cherry tomatoes, sliced in half

2 tablespoons fresh basil, minced

Directions

1. Preparing the Ingredients

Slice the ends off the cucumber (about ½ inch from each side) and slice the cucumber into 1-inch pieces. With a paring knife or a spoon, scoop most of the seeds from the inside of each cucumber piece to make a cup, being careful to not cut all the way through. Fill each cucumber cup with about 1 tablespoon of hummus or bean dip. Top each with a cherry tomato half and a sprinkle of fresh minced basil. Experiment with different toppings such as chopped olives, sun-dried tomatoes, or feta cheese instead of the cherry tomatoes and basil.

Eggplant Relish Spread

PREP TIME: 10 MINUTES / COOK TIME: 20 MINUTES/ MAKES ONE POT / SERVES 6

Ingredients

2 tablespoons extra-virgin olive oil

1 cup finely chopped onion (about ½ medium onion)

1 garlic clove, minced (about ½ teaspoon)

1 large globe eggplant, cut into ½-inch cubes (about 5 cups)

¼ teaspoon kosher or sea salt

1 (12-ounce) jar roasted red peppers, chopped
1½ cups chopped fresh tomatoes
½ cup balsamic or red wine vinegar
½ cup capers or chopped olives

Directions

1. Preparing the Ingredients

In a large skillet over medium heat, heat the oil.

Add the onion and cook for 4 minutes, stirring occasionally. Add the garlic and cook for 1 minute, stirring often. Turn up the heat to medium-high, and add the eggplant and salt. Cook for 5 minutes, stirring occasionally. Add the peppers, tomatoes, and vinegar, stir, and cover. Cook for 10 minutes, stirring every minute or so to prevent everything from sticking. If it looks like it's starting to stick and burn, turn down the heat to medium and add 1 tablespoon of water.

Remove from the heat, stir in the capers, and let sit for a few minutes to let the liquid absorb. Stir and serve, or store in a covered jar in the refrigerator for up to 10 days. It tastes even better the day after you make it!

Soups And Salads
Hearty Italian Turkey Vegetable Soup

PREP TIME: 30 MINUTES / COOK TIME: 1 HOUR 10 MINUTES / SERVES 2 WITH 2 SERVINGS FOR LEFTOVERS

Ingredients

1 tablespoon olive oil

½ pound lean ground turkey

1 celery stalk, diced (about ¼ cup)

2 medium carrots, diced (about ¾ cup)

1 small onion, diced (about 1 cup)

1 small fennel bulb, diced (about 1 cup)

1 garlic clove, minced

1 large leaf lacinato (dinosaur) kale, stemmed and chopped

2½ cups low-sodium tomato juice

2 cups low-sodium chicken stock

1 (15-ounce) can kidney beans, drained and rinsed

¾ teaspoon fennel seeds

¼ teaspoon red pepper flakes (optional)

¾ cup small shell pasta

2 tablespoons fresh basil, thinly sliced (about 4 basil leaves)

Salt

Directions

1. **Preparing the Ingredients**

Heat the olive oil in a stockpot over medium-high heat. Add the turkey and sauté for 10 minutes, or until it's no longer pink.

2. **Cooking**

Add the celery, carrots, onion, fennel, garlic, and kale and sauté for about 10 minutes. Add the tomato juice, chicken stock, kidney beans, fennel seeds, and red pepper flakes and bring the soup to a boil. Reduce the heat, cover the pot, and let the soup simmer for 40 minutes, or until the carrots are softened. Add the pasta and cook for another 10 minutes, or until al dente. Add the basil, and season with salt to taste—start with about ½ teaspoon.

Pistachio Parmesan Kale-Arugula Salad

PREP TIME: 20 MINUTES / COOK TIME: 10 MINUTES/ SERVES 6

Ingredients

6 cups raw kale, center ribs removed and discarded, leaves coarsely chopped

¼ cup extra-virgin olive oil

2 tablespoons freshly squeezed lemon juice (from about 1 small lemon)

½ teaspoon smoked paprika

2 cups arugula

⅓ cup unsalted shelled pistachios

6 tablespoons grated Parmesan or Pecorino Romano cheese

Directions

1. Preparing the Ingredients

In a large salad bowl, combine the kale, oil, lemon juice, and smoked paprika. With your hands, gently massage the leaves for about 15 seconds or so, until all are thoroughly coated. Let the kale sit for 10 minutes.

When you're ready to serve, gently mix in the arugula and pistachios. Divide the salad among six serving bowls, sprinkle 1 tablespoon of grated cheese over each, and serve.

Pistachio Quinoa Salad with Pomegranate Citrus Vinaigrette

PREP TIME: 15 MINUTES / COOK TIME: 15 MINUTES/ SERVES 6

Ingredients

1½ cups water
1 cup quinoa
¼ teaspoon kosher salt
1 cup extra-virgin olive oil
½ cup pomegranate juice
½ cup freshly squeezed orange juice
1 small shallot, minced
1 teaspoon pure maple syrup
1 teaspoon za'atar
½ teaspoon ground sumac
½ teaspoon kosher salt
¼ teaspoon freshly ground black pepper
3 cups baby spinach
½ cup fresh parsley, coarsely chopped
½ cup fresh mint, coarsely chopped
Approximately ¾ cup pomegranate seeds, or 2 pomegranates
¼ cup pistachios, shelled and toasted
¼ cup crumbled blue cheese

Directions

1. **Preparing the Ingredients**

Bring the water, quinoa, and salt to a boil in a small saucepan. Reduce the heat and cover; simmer for 10 to 12 minutes. Fluff with a fork. In a medium bowl, whisk together the olive oil, pomegranate juice, orange juice, shallot, maple syrup, za'atar, sumac, salt, and black pepper. In a large bowl, add about ½ cup of dressing.

Store the remaining dressing in a glass jar or airtight container and refrigerate.
The dressing can be kept up to 2 weeks.

Let the chilled dressing reach room temperature before using. Combine the spinach, parsley, and mint in the bowl with the dressing and toss gently together. Add the quinoa. Toss gently.

Add the pomegranate seeds. Or, if using whole pomegranates: Cut the pomegranates in half. Fill a large bowl with water and hold the pomegranate half, cut side-down. Using a wooden spoon, hit the back of the pomegranate so the seeds fall into the water. Immerse the pomegranate in the water and gently pull out any remaining seeds.

Repeat with the remaining pomegranate. Skim the white pith off the top of the water. Drain the seeds and add them to the greens. Add the pistachios and cheese and toss gently.

You can use any citrus juice you like for the dressing. Try lemon, lime, or grapefruit in place of orange.

Greek Salad

Ingredients

1 head romaine lettuce, torn
½ cup black olives, pitted and chopped
1 red onion, thinly sliced
1 tomato, chopped
1 cucumber, chopped
½ cup crumbled feta cheese
2 tablespoons extra-virgin olive oil
2 tablespoons red wine vinegar
Juice of 1 lemon
1 tablespoon dried oregano (or 2 tablespoons chopped fresh oregano leaves)
3 garlic cloves, minced
½ teaspoon Dijon mustard
½ teaspoon sea salt
¼ teaspoon freshly ground black pepper

Directions

1. Preparing the Ingredients

In a large bowl, mix the lettuce, olives, red onion, tomato, cucumber, and feta.

To make the dressing: In a small bowl, whisk the olive oil, vinegar, lemon juice, oregano, garlic, mustard, sea salt, and pepper.

Just before serving, toss the salad with the dressing.

Add 4 chopped hardboiled eggs to make this a hearty protein-filled meal.

Creamy Tomato Hummus Soup

PREP TIME: 10 MINUTES / COOK TIME: 10 MINUTES / SERVES 2 WITH 2 SERVINGS FOR LEFTOVERS

Ingredients

1 (14.5-ounce) can crushed tomatoes with basil

1 cup roasted red pepper hummus

2 cups low-sodium chicken stock

Salt

¼ cup fresh basil leaves, thinly sliced (optional, for garnish)

Garlic croutons (optional, for garnish)

Directions

Preparing the Ingredients

1. Combine the canned tomatoes, hummus, and chicken stock in a blender and blend until smooth. Pour the mixture into a saucepan and bring it to a boil.
Season with salt and fresh basil if desired. Serve with garlic croutons as a garnish, if desired.

2. To make this a heartier soup, add shredded chicken and precooked brown rice or barley.

Easy Italian Orange and Celery Salad

PREP TIME: 15 MINUTES / COOK TIME: NONE/ SERVES 6

Ingredients

3 celery stalks, including leaves, sliced diagonally into ½-inch slices

2 large oranges, peeled and sliced into rounds

½ cup green olives (or any variety)

¼ cup sliced red onion (about ¼ onion)

1 tablespoon extra-virgin olive oil

1 tablespoon olive brine

1 tablespoon freshly squeezed lemon or orange juice (from ½ small lemon or 1 orange round)

¼ teaspoon kosher or sea salt

¼ teaspoon freshly ground black pepper

Directions

Preparing the Ingredients

1. Place the celery, oranges, olives, and onion on a large serving platter or in a shallow, wide bowl.

2. In a small bowl, whisk together the oil, olive brine, and lemon juice. Pour over the salad, sprinkle with salt and pepper, and serve.

3. Instead of the orange rounds in this salad, you can swap in peeled and sectioned clementines or canned mandarin oranges in juice that have been drained.

Cauliflower Tabbouleh Salad

PREP TIME: 15 MINUTES / COOK TIME: 0 MINUTES / SERVES 4

Ingredients

¼ cup extra-virgin olive oil
¼ cup lemon juice
Zest of 1 lemon
¾ teaspoon kosher salt
½ teaspoon ground turmeric
¼ teaspoon ground coriander
¼ teaspoon ground cumin
¼ teaspoon black pepper
⅛ teaspoon ground cinnamon
1 pound riced cauliflower
1 English cucumber, diced
12 cherry tomatoes, halved
1 cup fresh parsley, chopped
½ cup fresh mint, chopped

Directions

Preparing the Ingredients

1. In a large bowl, whisk together the olive oil, lemon juice, lemon zest, salt, turmeric, coriander, cumin, black pepper, and cinnamon.
2. Add the riced cauliflower to the bowl and mix well. Add in the cucumber, tomatoes, parsley, and mint and gently mix together.

Cucumber Salad

Ingredients

4 medium cucumbers, chopped or spiralized into spaghetti noodles

1 tomato, chopped

3 scallions, white and green parts, chopped

2 tablespoons extra-virgin olive oil

¼ cup red wine vinegar

2 tablespoons chopped fresh dill

2 garlic cloves, minced

1 teaspoon Dijon mustard

½ teaspoon sea salt

¼ teaspoon freshly ground black pepper

Directions

Preparing the Ingredients

1. In a large bowl, mix together the cucumber, tomato, and scallions.

In a small bowl, whisk the olive oil, vinegar, dill, garlic, mustard, sea salt, and pepper.

Toss the dressing with the salad just before serving.

Cucumbers lend themselves nicely to various flavor profiles. To change things up, omit the tomato and add 3 more scallions.

2. For the dressing: Whisk 2 tablespoons extra-virgin olive oil, ¼ cup apple cider vinegar, 1 tablespoon grated fresh ginger, 3 minced garlic cloves, 2 tablespoons chopped fresh cilantro leaves, ½ teaspoon sea salt, and ⅛ teaspoon freshly ground black pepper.

Spicy Sausage Lentil Soup

Ingredients

1 tablespoon olive oil

½ medium onion, diced (about ¾ cup)

2 links (8 ounces) spicy Italian sausage (turkey or pork), removed from casing

2 medium carrots, sliced into coins (about ¾ cup)

1 medium celery stalk, diced (about ¼ cup)

2 garlic cloves, minced

¼ teaspoon red pepper flakes (omit or use less if you prefer less spicy)

½ teaspoon thyme

1 teaspoon oregano

1 bay leaf

3 cups low-sodium chicken stock

1 (28-ounce) can crushed tomatoes

¾ cup brown lentils

1 cup packed baby spinach, sliced

½ teaspoon salt, plus more to taste

Directions
Preparing the Ingredients

1. Heat the oil in a stockpot over medium-high heat. Add the onion and sausage and sauté, breaking up the sausage into small pieces.

Add the carrots, celery, and garlic, and continue to sauté for about 10 more minutes. Add the red pepper flakes, thyme, oregano, bay leaf, chicken stock, and tomatoes. Bring the soup to a boil.

2. Reduce the heat to medium-low and add the lentils. Stir everything well, cover, and let the soup simmer for 45 minutes, or until the lentils and carrots are tender.

Remove the bay leaf. Add the spinach and season with salt—start with ½ teaspoon and add additional salt to taste.

Spanish Style Turkey Meatball Soup (Instant Pot)

Ingredients

1 slice hearty white sandwich bread, torn into quarters
¼ cup whole milk
1 ounce Manchego cheese, grated (½ cup), plus extra for serving
5 tablespoons minced fresh parsley, divided
½ teaspoon table salt
1 pound ground turkey
1 tablespoon extra-virgin olive oil
1 onion, chopped
1 red bell pepper, stemmed, seeded, and cut into ¾-inch pieces
4 garlic cloves, minced
2 teaspoons smoked paprika
½ cup dry white wine
8 cups chicken broth
8 ounces kale, stemmed and chopped

Directions

Preparing the Ingredients

1. Using fork, mash bread and milk together into paste in large bowl. Stir in Manchego, 3 tablespoons parsley, and salt until combined. Add turkey and knead mixture with your hands until well combined. Pinch off and roll 2-teaspoon-size pieces of mixture into balls and arrange on large plate (you should have about 35 meatballs); set aside.

Using highest sauté function, heat oil in Instant Pot until shimmering. Add onion and bell pepper and cook until softened and lightly browned, 5 to 7 minutes. Stir in garlic and paprika and cook until fragrant, about 30 seconds. Stir in wine, scraping up any browned bits, and cook until almost completely evaporated, about 5 minutes. Stir in broth and kale, then gently submerge meatballs.

2. Lock lid in place and close pressure release valve. Select high pressure cook function and cook for 3 minutes. Turn off Instant Pot and quick-release pressure. Carefully remove lid, allowing steam to escape away from you.

3. Stir in remaining 2 tablespoons parsley and season with salt and pepper to taste. Serve, passing extra Manchego separately.

Melon Caprese Salad

Ingredients

1 cantaloupe, quartered and seeded
½ small seedless watermelon
1 cup grape tomatoes
2 cups fresh mozzarella balls (about 8 ounces)
⅓ cup fresh basil or mint leaves, torn into small pieces

2 tablespoons extra-virgin olive oil
1 tablespoon balsamic vinegar
¼ teaspoon freshly ground black pepper
¼ teaspoon kosher or sea salt

Directions

Preparing the Ingredients

1. Using a melon baller or a metal, teaspoon-size measuring spoon, scoop balls out of the cantaloupe. You should get about 2½ to 3 cups from one cantaloupe. (If you prefer, cut the melon into bite-size pieces instead of making balls.) Put them in a large colander over a large serving bowl.

2. Using the same method, ball or cut the watermelon into bite-size pieces; you should get about 2 cups. Put the watermelon balls in the colander with the cantaloupe.

3. Let the fruit drain for 10 minutes. Pour the juice from the bowl into a container to refrigerate and save for drinking or adding to smoothies. Wipe the bowl dry, and put in the cut fruit.

4. Add the tomatoes, mozzarella, basil, oil, vinegar, pepper, and salt to the fruit mixture. Gently mix until everything is incorporated and serve.

If you want to make this recipe a day ahead, prepare the salad through step 3. Cover and refrigerate. Before serving, drain the fruit again for about 5 minutes. Add it back into the serving bowl, then toss it with the remaining ingredients.

Caprese Salad

PREP TIME: 15 MINUTES / COOK TIME: NONE / SERVES 4

Ingredients

3 large tomatoes, sliced

4 ounces part-skim mozzarella cheese, cut into ¼-inch-thick slices

¼ cup balsamic vinegar

2 tablespoons extra-virgin olive oil

½ teaspoon sea salt

¼ cup loosely packed basil leaves, torn

Directions

Preparing the Ingredients

1. On a pretty platter, arrange the tomatoes and cheese slices alternating and overlapping in a row.

Drizzle with the vinegar and olive oil.

Sprinkle with sea salt and basil and serve.

2. Replace the balsamic vinegar with an equal amount of freshly squeezed lemon juice or red wine vinegar.

Vegetable Fagioli

PREP TIME: 30 MINUTES / COOK TIME: 60 MINUTES / SERVES 2 WITH 2 SERVINGS FOR LEFTOVERS

Ingredients

1 tablespoon olive oil

2 medium carrots, diced (about ¾ cup)

2 medium celery stalks, diced (about ½ cup)

½ medium onion, diced (about ¾ cup)

1 large garlic clove, minced

3 tablespoons tomato paste

4 cups low-sodium vegetable broth

1 cup packed kale, stemmed and chopped

1 (15-ounce) can red kidney beans, drained and rinsed

1 (15-ounce) can cannellini beans, drained and rinsed

½ cup fresh basil, chopped

Salt

Freshly ground black pepper

Directions

Preparing the Ingredients

1. Heat the olive oil in a stockpot over medium-high heat. Add the carrots, celery, onion, and garlic and sauté for 10 minutes, or until the vegetables start to turn golden.

Stir in the tomato paste and cook for about 30 seconds.

2. Add the vegetable broth and bring the soup to a boil. Cover, and reduce the heat to low. Cook the soup for 45 minutes, or until the carrots are tender.

3. Using an immersion blender, purée the soup so that it's partly smooth, but with some chunks of vegetables. If you don't have an immersion blender, scoop out about ⅓ of the soup and blend it in a blender, then add it back to the pot.

Add the kale, beans, and basil. Season with salt and pepper.

Classic Chicken Broth

PREP TIME: 15 MINUTES / COOK TIME: 30 MINUTES/ MAKES: 8 CUPS / SERVES 4

Ingredients

4 pounds chicken backs and wings

14 cups water

1 onion, chopped

2 bay leaves

2 teaspoons salt

Directions

1. Heat chicken and water in large stockpot or Dutch oven over medium-high heat until boiling, skimming off any scum that comes to surface. Reduce heat to low and simmer gently for 3 hours.

Add onion, bay leaves, and salt and continue to simmer for another 2 hours.

2. Strain broth through fine-mesh strainer into large pot or container, pressing on solids to extract as much liquid as possible. Let broth settle for about 5 minutes, then skim off fat. (Cooled broth can be refrigerated for up to 4 days or frozen for up to 1 month.)

Beef Oxtail Soup with White Beans, Tomatoes, and Aleppo Pepper (Instant Pot)

PREP TIME: 10 MINUTES / COOK TIME: 1 HOUR / SERVES 6 TO 8

Ingredients

4 pounds oxtails, trimmed

1 teaspoon table salt

1 tablespoon extra-virgin olive oil

1 onion, chopped fine

2 carrots, peeled and chopped fine

¼ cup ground dried Aleppo pepper

6 garlic cloves, minced

2 tablespoons tomato paste

¾ teaspoon dried oregano

½ teaspoon ground cinnamon

½ teaspoon ground cumin

6 cups water

1 (28-ounce) can diced tomatoes, drained

1 (15-ounce) can navy beans, rinsed

1 tablespoon sherry vinegar

¼ cup chopped fresh parsley

½ preserved lemon, pulp and white pith removed, rind rinsed and minced (2 tablespoons)

Directions

Preparing the Ingredients

1. Pat oxtails dry with paper towels and sprinkle with salt. Using highest sauté function, heat oil in Instant Pot for 5 minutes (or until just smoking). Brown half of oxtails, 4 to 6 minutes per side; transfer to plate. Set aside remaining uncooked oxtails.

2. Add onion and carrots to fat left in pot and cook, using highest sauté function, until softened, about 5 minutes. Stir in Aleppo pepper, garlic, tomato paste, oregano, cinnamon, and cumin and cook until fragrant, about 30 seconds. Stir in water, scraping up any browned bits, then stir in tomatoes. Nestle remaining uncooked oxtails into pot along with browned oxtails and add any accumulated juices.

3. Lock lid in place and close pressure release valve. Select high pressure cook function and cook for 45 minutes. Turn off Instant Pot and quick-release pressure. Carefully remove lid, allowing steam to escape away from you.

4. Transfer oxtails to cutting board, let cool slightly, then shred into bite-size pieces using 2 forks; discard bones and excess fat. Strain broth through fine-mesh strainer into large container; return solids to now-empty pot. Using wide, shallow spoon, skim excess fat from surface of liquid; return to pot.

5. Stir shredded oxtails and any accumulated juices and beans into pot. Using highest sauté function, cook until soup is heated through, about 5 minutes. Stir

in vinegar and parsley and season with salt and pepper to taste. Serve, passing preserved lemon separately.

Chopped Greek Antipasto Salad

PREP TIME: 20 MINUTES / COOK TIME: NONE / SERVES 6

Ingredients

1 head Bibb lettuce or ½ head romaine lettuce, chopped (about 2½ cups)

¼ cup loosely packed chopped basil leaves

1 (15-ounce) can chickpeas, drained and rinsed

1 (14-ounce) can artichoke hearts, drained and halved

1 pint grape tomatoes, halved (about 1½ cups)

1 seedless cucumber, peeled and chopped (about 1½ cups)

½ cup cubed feta cheese (about 2 ounces)

1 (2.25-ounce) can sliced black olives (about ½ cup)

For the dressing

3 tablespoons extra-virgin olive oil

1 tablespoon red wine vinegar

1 tablespoon freshly squeezed lemon juice (from about ½ small lemon)

1 tablespoon chopped fresh oregano or ½ teaspoon dried oregano

1 teaspoon honey

¼ teaspoon freshly ground black pepper

Directions

Preparing the Ingredients

1. In a medium bowl, toss the lettuce and basil together. Spread out on a large serving platter or in a large salad bowl. Arrange the chickpeas, artichoke hearts, tomatoes, cucumber, feta, and olives in piles next to each other on top of the lettuce layer.

2. In a small pitcher or bowl, whisk together the oil, vinegar, lemon juice, oregano, honey, and pepper. Serve on the side with the salad, or drizzle over all the ingredients right before serving.

3. Take this dressing to the next level and make a quick oregano oil infusion. Put the oil and oregano in a small skillet over medium-low heat. Let it cook for 5 minutes, stirring occasionally. Remove from the heat and strain through a fine mesh strainer.

Roasted Golden Beet, Avocado, and Watercress Salad

PREP TIME: 15 MINUTES / COOK TIME: 1 HOUR/ SERVES 4

Ingredients

1 bunch (about 1½ pounds) golden beets

1 tablespoon extra-virgin olive oil

1 tablespoon white wine vinegar

½ teaspoon kosher salt

¼ teaspoon freshly ground black pepper

1 bunch (about 4 ounces) watercress

1 avocado, peeled, pitted, and diced

¼ cup crumbled feta cheese

¼ cup walnuts, toasted

1 tablespoon fresh chives, chopped

Directions

Preparing the Ingredients

1. Preheat the oven to 425°F. Wash and trim the beets (cut an inch above the beet root, leaving the long tail if desired), then wrap each beet individually in foil. Place the beets on a baking sheet and roast until fully cooked, 45 to 60 minutes depending on the size of each beet. Start checking at 45 minutes; if easily pierced with a fork, the beets are cooked.

2. Remove the beets from the oven and allow them to cool. Under cold running water, slough off the skin. Cut the beets into bite-size cubes or wedges.

3. In a large bowl, whisk together the olive oil, vinegar, salt, and black pepper. Add the watercress and beets and toss well. Add the avocado, feta, walnuts, and chives and mix gently.

Mediterranean Potato Salad

PREP TIME: 10 MINUTES / COOK TIME: 20 MINUTES/ SERVES 6

Ingredients

2 pounds Yukon Gold baby potatoes, cut into 1-inch cubes

3 tablespoons freshly squeezed lemon juice (from about 1 medium lemon)

3 tablespoons extra-virgin olive oil

1 tablespoon olive brine

¼ teaspoon kosher or sea salt

1 (2.25-ounce) can sliced olives (about ½ cup)

1 cup sliced celery (about 2 stalks) or fennel

2 tablespoons chopped fresh oregano

2 tablespoons torn fresh mint

Directions

Preparing the Ingredients

1. In a medium saucepan, cover the potatoes with cold water until the waterline is one inch above the potatoes. Set over high heat, bring the potatoes to a boil, then turn down the heat to medium-low. Simmer for 12 to 15 minutes, until the potatoes are just fork tender.

While the potatoes are cooking, in a small bowl, whisk together the lemon juice, oil, olive brine, and salt.

2. Drain the potatoes in a colander and transfer to a serving bowl. Immediately pour about 3 tablespoons of the dressing over the potatoes. Gently mix in the olives and celery.

3. Before serving, gently mix in the oregano, mint, and the remaining dressing.

Wild Rice Salad with Chickpeas and Pickled Radish

PREP TIME: 20 MINUTES / COOK TIME: 45 MINUTES/ SERVES 4

Ingredients

1 cup water

4 ounces (⅔ cup) wild rice

¼ teaspoon kosher salt

1 bunch radishes (6 to 8 small), sliced thin

½ cup white wine vinegar

½ teaspoon kosher salt

2 tablespoons extra-virgin olive oil

2 tablespoons white wine vinegar

½ teaspoon pure maple syrup

½ teaspoon kosher salt

¼ teaspoon freshly ground black pepper

1 (15-ounce) can no-salt-added or low-sodium chickpeas, rinsed and drained

1 bulb fennel, diced

¼ cup walnuts, chopped and toasted

¼ cup crumbled feta cheese

¼ cup currants

2 tablespoons fresh dill, chopped

Directions

Preparing the Ingredients

1. Bring the water, rice, and salt to a boil in a medium saucepan. Cover, reduce the heat, and simmer for 45 minutes.
2. In a medium bowl, combine the radishes, vinegar, and salt. Let sit for 15 to 30 minutes.

In a large bowl, whisk together the olive oil, vinegar, maple syrup, salt, and black pepper. While still warm, add the rice to the bowl with the dressing and mix well.

3. Add the chickpeas, fennel, walnuts, feta, currants, and dill. Mix well.

Garnish with the pickled radishes before serving.

Chop Chop Salad

PREP TIME: 15 MINUTES / COOK TIME: NONE/ SERVES 6

Ingredients

2 heads romaine lettuce, chopped

3 cups chopped skinless cooked chicken breast

1 cup canned or jarred (in water) artichoke hearts, drained, rinsed, and chopped

2 tomatoes, chopped

2 zucchini, chopped

½ red onion, finely chopped

3 ounces mozzarella cheese, chopped

⅓ cup unsweetened nonfat plain Greek yogurt

1 tablespoon Dijon mustard

2 tablespoons extra-virgin olive oil

Zest of 1 lemon

3 garlic cloves, minced

2 tablespoons chopped fresh basil leaves

2 tablespoons chopped fresh chives

½ teaspoon sea salt

⅛ teaspoon freshly ground black pepper

Directions

Preparing the Ingredients

1. In a large bowl, combine the lettuce, chicken, artichoke hearts, tomatoes, zucchini, red onion, and mozzarella.
2. In a small bowl, whisk the yogurt, mustard, olive oil, lemon zest, garlic, basil, chives, sea salt, and pepper.

Toss the dressing with the salad before serving.

Fig and Arugula Salad

PREP TIME: 15 MINUTES / COOK TIME: 30 MINUTES / SERVES 2

Ingredients

3 cups arugula

4 fresh, ripe figs (or 4 to 6 dried figs), stemmed and sliced

2 tablespoons olive oil

3 very thin slices prosciutto, trimmed of any fat and sliced lengthwise into 1-inch strips

¼ cup pecan halves, lightly toasted

2 tablespoons crumbled blue cheese

1 to 2 tablespoons balsamic glaze

Directions

Preparing the Ingredients

1. In a large bowl, toss the arugula and figs with the olive oil.
2. Place the prosciutto on a microwave-safe plate and heat it on high in the microwave for 60 seconds, or until it just starts to crisp.

Add the crisped prosciutto, pecans, and blue cheese to the bowl. Toss the salad lightly.

3. Drizzle with the balsamic glaze.

Quinoa with Zucchini, Mint, and Pistachios

PREP TIME: 20 TO 30 MINUTES / COOK TIME: 20 MINUTES/ SERVES 4

Ingredients

1½ cups water

1 cup quinoa

¼ teaspoon kosher salt

2 tablespoons extra-virgin olive oil

1 zucchini, thinly sliced into rounds

6 small radishes, sliced

1 shallot, julienned

¾ teaspoon kosher salt

¼ teaspoon freshly ground black pepper

2 garlic cloves, sliced

61

Zest of 1 lemon

2 tablespoons lemon juice

¼ cup fresh mint, chopped

¼ cup fresh basil, chopped

¼ cup pistachios, shelled and toasted

Directions

Preparing the Ingredients. Bring the water, quinoa, and salt to a boil in a medium saucepan. Reduce to a simmer, cover, and cook for 10 to 12 minutes. Fluff with a fork. Heat the olive oil in a large skillet or sauté pan over medium-high heat. Add the zucchini, radishes, shallot, salt, and black pepper, and sauté for 7 to 8 minutes. Add the garlic and cook 30 seconds to 1 minute more. In a large bowl, combine the lemon zest and lemon juice. Add the quinoa and mix well. Add the cooked zucchini mixture and mix well. Add the mint, basil, and pistachios and gently mix.

Panzanella

PREP TIME: 15 MINUTES / COOK TIME: 8 MINUTES/ SERVES 4

Ingredients

6 tablespoons extra-virgin olive oil, divided

4 whole-grain bread slices, crusts removed, cut into pieces

1 cup yellow cherry tomatoes, halved

1 cup red cherry tomatoes, halved

1 plum tomato, cut into wedges

½ red onion, very thinly sliced

¼ cup chopped fresh basil leaves

1 tablespoon capers, drained and rinsed

¼ cup red wine vinegar

2 garlic cloves, minced

½ teaspoon Dijon mustard

½ teaspoon sea salt

¼ teaspoon freshly ground black pepper

Directions

Preparing the Ingredients. In a large skillet over medium-high heat, heat 2 tablespoons of olive oil until it shimmers.

Add the bread and cook for 6 to 8 minutes, stirring occasionally, until crisp and browned. Drain and cool the bread on paper towels. In a large bowl, combine the cooled bread, yellow, red, and plum tomatoes, red onion, basil, and capers. In a small bowl, whisk the remaining 4 tablespoons of olive oil with the vinegar, garlic, mustard, sea salt, and pepper. Toss with the salad and serve.

Summer Panzanella Salad

PREP TIME: 15 MINUTES / COOK TIME: 10 MINUTES, PLUS 15 MINUTES TO REST / SERVES 2

Ingredients

1 ear corn on the cob, peeled and shucked

4 slices stale French baguette

½ pint cherry or grape tomatoes, halved
1 medium sweet pepper, seeded and cut into 1-inch pieces
1 medium avocado, pitted and cut into cubes
4 very thin slices of sweet onion, cut crosswise into thin rings
½ cup fresh whole basil leaves
2 ounces mini mozzarella balls (ciliegine), halved or quartered
¼ cup honey balsamic dressing
Cooking spray

Directions

Preparing the Ingredients

1. Heat the grill to medium-high heat (about 350°F) and lightly spray the cooking grates with cooking spray.
2. Grill the corn for 10 minutes, or until it is lightly charred all around. Grill the bread for 30 to 45 seconds on each side, or until it has grill marks. Let the corn sit until it's cool enough to handle. Cut the kernels off the cob and place them in a large bowl. Cut the bread into chunks and add it to the bowl.
3. Add the tomatoes, sweet pepper, avocado, onion, basil, mozzarella, and dressing to the bowl, and toss lightly to combine. Let the salad sit for about 15 minutes in the refrigerator, so the bread can soften and the flavors can blend.

This is best served shortly after it's prepared.

Sicilian Fish Stew(Instant Pot)

PREP TIME: 23 MINUTES / COOK TIME: 22 MINUTES/ SERVES 4 TO 6

Ingredients
2 tablespoons extra-virgin olive oil
2 onions, chopped fine
1 teaspoon table salt
½ teaspoon pepper
1 teaspoon minced fresh thyme or ¼ teaspoon dried
Pinch red pepper flakes
4 garlic cloves, minced, divided
1 (28-ounce) can whole peeled tomatoes, drained with juice reserved, chopped coarse
1 (8-ounce) bottle clam juice
¼ cup dry white wine
¼ cup golden raisins
2 tablespoons capers, rinsed
1½ pounds skinless swordfish steak, 1 to 1½ inches thick, cut into 1-inch pieces
¼ cup pine nuts, toasted
¼ cup minced fresh mint
1 teaspoon grated orange zest

Directions

1. Using highest sauté function, heat oil in Instant Pot until shimmering. Add onions, salt, and pepper and cook until onions are softened, about 5 minutes.

Stir in thyme, pepper flakes, and three-quarters of garlic and cook until fragrant, about 30 seconds. Stir in tomatoes and reserved juice, clam juice, wine, raisins, and capers. Nestle swordfish into pot and spoon some cooking liquid over top.

2. Lock lid in place and close pressure release valve. Select high pressure cook function and cook for 1 minute. Turn off Instant Pot and quick-release pressure. Carefully remove lid, allowing steam to escape away from you.

3. Combine pine nuts, mint, orange zest, and remaining garlic in bowl. Season stew with salt and pepper to taste. Sprinkle individual portions with pine nut mixture before serving.

Pastina Chicken soup with kale

PREP TIME: 5 MINUTES / COOK TIME: 25 MINUTES/ MAKES 3 CUPS / SERVES 6

Ingredients

1 tablespoon extra-virgin olive oil
2 garlic cloves, minced (about 1 teaspoon)
3 cups packed chopped kale (center ribs removed)
1 cup minced carrots (about 2 carrots)
8 cups low-sodium or no-salt-added chicken (or vegetable) broth
¼ teaspoon kosher or sea salt
¼ teaspoon freshly ground black pepper
¾ cup (6 ounces) uncooked acini de pepe or pastina pasta
2 cups shredded cooked chicken (about 12 ounces)
3 tablespoons grated Parmesan cheese

Directions

1. **Preparing the Ingredients.** In a large stockpot over medium heat, heat the oil. Add the garlic and cook for 30 seconds, stirring frequently. Add the kale and carrots and cook for 5 minutes, stirring occasionally.

2. Add the broth, salt, and pepper, and turn the heat to high. Bring the broth to a boil, and add the pasta. Lower the heat to medium and cook for 10 minutes, or until the pasta is cooked through, stirring every few minutes so the pasta doesn't stick to the bottom. Add the chicken, and cook for 2 more minutes to warm through.

Ladle the soup into six bowls, top each with ½ tablespoon of cheese, and serve.

Italian White Bean Salad with Bell Peppers

PREP TIME: 15 MINUTES / COOK TIME: 20 MINUTES / SERVES 4

Ingredients

2 tablespoons extra-virgin olive oil
2 tablespoons white wine vinegar
½ shallot, minced
½ teaspoon kosher salt
¼ teaspoon freshly ground black pepper
3 cups cooked cannellini beans, or 2 (15-ounce) cans no-salt-added or low-sodium cannellini beans, drained and rinsed

2 celery stalks, diced

½ red bell pepper, diced

¼ cup fresh parsley, chopped

¼ cup fresh mint, chopped

Directions

Preparing the Ingredients

1. In a large bowl, whisk together the olive oil, vinegar, shallot, salt, and black pepper.
2. Add the beans, celery, red bell pepper, parsley, and mint; mix well.

To make this salad a heartier lunch or dinner, mix in a cooked whole grain such as farro or sorghum.

Simple Summer Gazpacho

PREP TIME: 15 MINUTES (PLUS 1 HOUR TO CHILL) / COOK TIME: NONE/ SERVES 4

Ingredients

6 tomatoes, chopped

3 garlic cloves, minced

2 red bell peppers, finely chopped

1 red onion, finely chopped

3 cups tomato juice

¼ cup red wine vinegar

¼ cup extra-virgin olive oil

¼ cup basil leaves, torn

½ teaspoon sea salt

¼ teaspoon freshly ground black pepper

Directions

1. In a blender or food processor, combine the tomatoes, garlic, red bell peppers, red onion, tomato juice, vinegar, olive oil, basil, sea salt, and pepper. Pulse for 20 to 30 (1-second) pulses until blended. Chill for 1 hour before serving.
2. Spice it up by adding 1 chile pepper or a few dashes of your favorite hot sauce.

Watermelon Feta Salad

PREP TIME: 10 MINUTES / COOK TIME: NONE/ MAKES 3 CUPS / SERVES 2

Ingredients

3 cups packed arugula

2½ cups watermelon, cut into bite-size cubes

2 ounces feta cheese, crumbled

2 tablespoons balsamic glaze

Directions

Preparing the Ingredients

1. Divide the arugula between two plates. Divide the watermelon cubes between the beds of arugula. Sprinkle 1 ounce of the feta over each salad.
2. Drizzle about 1 tablespoon of the glaze (or more if desired) over each salad.

Roasted Red Pepper Soup with Smoked Paprika and Cilantro Yogurt

PREP TIME: 15 MINUTES / COOK TIME: 10 MINUTES/ SERVES 6

Ingredients

½ cup whole-milk yogurt

3 tablespoons minced fresh cilantro

1 teaspoon lime juice

Salt and pepper

8 red bell peppers, cored and flattened

1 tablespoon extra-virgin olive oil

2 garlic cloves, minced

1 red onion, chopped

½ teaspoon ground cumin

½ teaspoon smoked paprika

2 tablespoons tomato paste

1 tablespoon all-purpose flour

4 cups chicken or vegetable broth, plus extra as needed

1 bay leaf

½ cup half-and-half

2 tablespoons dry sherry

Directions

Preparing the Ingredients

1. Whisk yogurt, 1 tablespoon cilantro, and lime juice together in bowl. Season with salt and pepper to taste. Cover and refrigerate until needed.
2. Adjust oven rack 3 inches from broiler element and heat broiler. Spread half of peppers skin side up on aluminum foil–lined baking sheet. Broil until skin is charred and puffed but flesh is still firm, 8 to 10 minutes, rotating sheet halfway through broiling. Transfer broiled peppers to bowl, cover with plastic wrap or

foil, and let steam until skins peel off easily, 10 to 15 minutes. Repeat with remaining peppers. Peel broiled peppers, discarding skins, and chop coarse.

3. Cook oil and garlic together in Dutch oven over low heat, stirring constantly, until garlic is foamy, sticky, and straw-colored, 6 to 8 minutes. Stir in onion and ¼ teaspoon salt, increase heat to medium, and cook until softened, about 5 minutes.

4. Stir in cumin and paprika and cook until fragrant, about 30 seconds. Stir in tomato paste and flour and cook for 1 minute. Slowly whisk in broth, scraping up any browned bits and smoothing out any lumps. Stir in bay leaf and chopped peppers, bring to simmer, and cook until peppers are very tender, 5 to 7 minutes.

5. Discard bay leaf. Working in batches, process soup in blender until smooth, about 2 minutes. Return soup to clean pot and stir in half- and-half and sherry. Heat soup gently over low heat until hot (do not boil) and adjust consistency with extra hot broth as needed. Stir in remaining 2 tablespoons cilantro and season with salt and pepper to taste. Serve, drizzling individual portions with yogurt mixture.

Mushroom Barley Soup

Ingredients

2 tablespoons extra-virgin olive oil

1 cup chopped onion (about ½ medium onion)

1 cup chopped carrots (about 2 carrots)

5½ cups chopped mushrooms (about 12 ounces)

6 cups low-sodium or no-salt-added vegetable broth

1 cup uncooked pearled barley

¼ cup red wine

2 tablespoons tomato paste

4 sprigs fresh thyme or ½ teaspoon dried thyme

1 dried bay leaf

6 tablespoons grated Parmesan cheese

Directions

Preparing the Ingredients

1. In a large stockpot over medium heat, heat the oil. Add the onion and carrots and cook for 5 minutes, stirring frequently. Turn up the heat to medium-high and add the mushrooms. Cook for 3 minutes, stirring frequently.
2. Add the broth, barley, wine, tomato paste, thyme, and bay leaf. Stir, cover the pot, and bring the soup to a boil. Once it's boiling, stir a few times, reduce the heat to medium-low, cover, and cook for another 12 to 15 minutes, until the barley is cooked through.

Remove the bay leaf and serve in soup bowls with 1 tablespoon of cheese sprinkled on top of each.

French Lentil Salad with Parsley and Mint

Ingredients

1 cup French lentils

1 garlic clove, smashed

1 dried bay leaf

2 tablespoons extra-virgin olive oil

2 tablespoons red wine vinegar

½ teaspoon ground cumin

½ teaspoon kosher salt

¼ teaspoon freshly ground black pepper

2 celery stalks, diced small

1 bell pepper, diced small

½ red onion, diced small

¼ cup fresh parsley, chopped

¼ cup fresh mint, chopped

Directions

Preparing the Ingredients

1. Put the lentils, garlic, and bay leaf in a large saucepan. Cover with water by about 3 inches and bring to a boil. Reduce the heat, cover, and simmer until tender, 20 to 30 minutes.
2. Drain the lentils to remove any remaining water after cooking. Remove the garlic and bay leaf.
3. In a large bowl, whisk together the olive oil, vinegar, cumin, salt, and black pepper. Add the celery, bell pepper, onion, parsley, and mint and toss to combine. Add the lentils and mix well.

Butternut Squash Soup

PREP TIME: 15 MINUTES / COOK TIME: 35 MINUTES/ MAKES 4 CUPS / SERVES 4

Ingredients

2 tablespoons extra-virgin olive oil

1 onion, chopped

1 carrot, chopped

1 celery stalk, chopped

4 cups unsalted vegetable broth

3 cups chopped butternut squash

1 teaspoon dried thyme

½ teaspoon sea salt

¼ teaspoon freshly ground black pepper

Directions

Preparing the Ingredients

1. In a large pot over medium-high heat, heat the olive oil until it shimmers. Add the onion, carrot, and celery. Cook for 5 to 7 minutes, stirring occasionally, until the vegetables begin to brown. Add the broth, squash, thyme, sea salt, and pepper. Bring to a simmer and reduce the heat to medium. Simmer for 20 to 30 minutes until the squash is soft.
2. Purée the soup using an immersion blender, food processor, or blender.

Easy Pasta Fagioli Soup

PREP TIME: 5 MINUTES / COOK TIME: 25 MINUTES/ SERVES 6

Ingredients

2 tablespoons extra-virgin olive oil

½ cup chopped onion (about ¼ onion)

3 garlic cloves, minced (about 1½ teaspoons)

1 tablespoon minced fresh rosemary or 1 teaspoon dried rosemary

¼ teaspoon crushed red pepper

4 cups low-sodium or no-salt-added vegetable broth

2 (15.5-ounce) cans cannellini, great northern, or light kidney beans, undrained

1 (28-ounce) can low-sodium or no-salt-added crushed tomatoes

2 tablespoons tomato paste

8 ounces uncooked short pasta, such as ditalini, tubetti, or elbows

6 tablespoons grated Parmesan cheese (about 1½ ounces)

Directions

1. In a large stockpot over medium heat, heat the oil. Add the onion and cook for 4 minutes, stirring frequently. Add the garlic, rosemary, and crushed red pepper. Cook for 1 minute, stirring frequently. Add the broth, canned beans with their liquid, tomatoes, and tomato paste. Simmer for 5 minutes.
2. To thicken the soup, carefully transfer 2 cups to a blender. Purée, then stir it back into the pot.
3. Bring the soup to a boil over high heat. Mix in the pasta, and lower the heat to a simmer. Cook the pasta for the amount of time recommended on the box, stirring every few minutes to prevent the pasta from sticking to the pot. Taste the pasta to make sure it is cooked through (it could take a few more minutes than the recommended cooking time, since it's cooking with other ingredients).
4. Ladle the soup into bowls, top each with 1 tablespoon of grated cheese, and serve.

Roasted Cauliflower and Arugula Salad with Pomegranate and Pine Nuts

PREP TIME: 5 MINUTES / COOK TIME: 20 MINUTES/ SERVES 4

Ingredients

1 head cauliflower, trimmed and cut into 1-inch florets

2 tablespoons extra-virgin olive oil, plus more for drizzling (optional)

1 teaspoon ground cumin

½ teaspoon kosher salt

¼ teaspoon freshly ground black pepper

5 ounces arugula

⅓ cup pomegranate seeds

¼ cup pine nuts, toasted

Directions

1. **Preparing the Ingredients**

Preheat the oven to 425°F. Line a baking sheet with parchment paper or foil. In a large bowl, combine the cauliflower, olive oil, cumin, salt, and black pepper.

2. **Cooking**

Spread in a single layer on the prepared baking sheet and roast for 20 minutes, tossing halfway through. Divide the arugula among 4 plates. Top with the cauliflower, pomegranate seeds, and pine nuts. Serve with Lemon Vinaigrette dressing or a simple drizzle of olive oil.

White Bean Soup with Kale

PREP TIME: 5 MINUTES / COOK TIME: 20 MINUTES/ SERVES 6

Ingredients

2 tablespoons extra-virgin olive oil

8 ounces Italian chicken sausage (uncooked), sliced

1 onion, chopped 1 carrot, chopped

1 red bell pepper, seeded and chopped

3 garlic cloves, minced

6 cups unsalted vegetable broth

1 (14-ounce) can white beans, drained

4 cups chopped kale

1 teaspoon dried thyme

½ teaspoon sea salt

¼ teaspoon freshly ground black pepper

Pinch red pepper flakes

Directions

Preparing the Ingredients

1. In a large pot over medium-high heat, heat the olive oil until it shimmers.
2. Add the sausage and cook for about 5 minutes, stirring occasionally, until browned. Remove the sausage from the pot with a slotted spoon and set it aside.

Add the onion, carrot, and red bell pepper to the oil remaining in the pot. Cook for about 5 minutes, stirring occasionally, until the vegetables are soft.

Add the garlic and cook for 30 seconds, stirring constantly.

3. Stir in the broth, beans, kale, thyme, sea salt, pepper, and red pepper flakes. Bring to a simmer. Reduce the heat to low and simmer for about 5 minutes more until the kale is soft.

Return the sausage to the pot. Cook for 1 minute more until the sausage heats through. Serve immediately.

Citrus Fennel Salad

PREP TIME: 15 MINUTES / COOK TIME: 0 MINUTES/ SERVES 2

Ingredients

2 tablespoons fresh orange juice

3 tablespoons olive oil

1 tablespoon blood orange vinegar, other orange vinegar, or cider vinegar

1 tablespoon honey

Salt

Freshly ground black pepper

For the salad

2 cups packed baby kale

1 medium navel or blood orange, segmented

½ small fennel bulb, stems and leaves removed, sliced into matchsticks

3 tablespoons toasted pecans, chopped

2 ounces goat cheese, crumbled
Directions

1. Preparing the Ingredients

Divide the baby kale, orange segments, fennel, pecans, and goat cheese evenly between two plates. Drizzle half of the dressing over each salad. Baby kale is usually sold prewashed in bags. If it's only available mixed with other greens, That works fine. Combine the orange juice, olive oil, vinegar, and honey in a small bowl and whisk to combine. Season with salt and pepper. Set the dressing aside.

Roasted Carrot Soup with Parmesan Croutons

PREP TIME: 10 MINUTES / COOK TIME: 20 MINUTES/ SERVES 4

Ingredients

2 pounds carrots, unpeeled, cut into ½-inch slices (about 6 cups)

2 tablespoons extra-virgin olive oil, divided

1 cup chopped onion (about ½ medium onion)

2 cups low-sodium or no-salt-added vegetable (or chicken) broth

2½ cups water

1 teaspoon dried thyme

¼ teaspoon crushed red pepper

¼ teaspoon kosher or sea salt

4 thin slices whole-grain bread

⅓ cup freshly grated Parmesan cheese (about 1 ounce)

Directions

1. Preparing the Ingredients

Place one oven rack about four inches below the broiler element. Place two large, rimmed baking sheets in the oven on any oven rack. Preheat the oven to 450°F.

2. Cooking

In a large bowl, toss the carrots with 1 tablespoon of oil to coat. With oven mitts, carefully remove the baking sheets from the oven and evenly distribute the carrots on both sheets. Bake for 20 minutes, until the carrots are just fork tender, stirring once halfway through. The carrots will still be somewhat firm. Remove the carrots from the oven, and turn the oven to the high broil setting. While the carrots are roasting, in a large stockpot over medium-high heat, heat 1 tablespoon of oil. Add the onion and cook for 5 minutes, stirring occasionally. Add the broth, water, thyme, crushed red pepper, and salt. Bring to a boil, cover, then remove the pan from the heat until the carrots have finished roasting.

Add the roasted carrots to the pot, and blend with an immersion blender (or use a regular blender—carefully pour in the hot soup in batches, then return the soup to the pot). Heat the soup for about 1 minute over medium-high heat, until warmed through. Turn the oven to the high broil setting. Place the bread on the baking sheet. Sprinkle the cheese evenly across the slices of bread. Broil the bread 4 inches below the heating element for 1 to 2 minutes, or until the cheese melts, watching carefully to prevent burning. Cut the bread into bite-size croutons. Divide the soup evenly among four bowls, top each with the Parmesan croutons, and serve.

Red Gazpacho

PREP TIME: 15 MINUTES / COOK TIME: 0 MINUTES/ SERVES 4

Ingredients

2 pounds tomatoes, cut into chunks

1 bell pepper, cut into chunks

1 cucumber, cut into chunks

1 small red onion, cut into chunks

1 garlic clove, smashed
2 teaspoons sherry vinegar
½ teaspoon kosher salt
¼ teaspoon freshly ground black pepper
⅓ cup extra-virgin olive oil
Lemon juice (optional)
¼ cup fresh chives, chopped, for garnish

Directions

Preparing the Ingredients

In a high-speed blender or Vitamix, add the tomatoes, bell pepper, cucumber, onion, garlic, vinegar, salt, and black pepper. Blend until smooth. With the motor running, add the olive oil and purée until smooth. Add more vinegar or a spritz of lemon juice if needed. Garnish with the chives. Any herbs will go nicely with this refreshing cold soup. Use parsley, basil, or whatever you like in place of the chives.

Lentil Soup

Ingredients

2 tablespoons extra-virgin olive oil

2 onions, chopped

2 celery stalks, chopped

2 carrots, chopped

4 garlic cloves, minced

1 (14-ounce) can lentils, drained

2 bay leaves

6 cups unsalted vegetable broth

1 teaspoon sea salt

¼ teaspoon freshly ground black pepper

Pinch red pepper flakes

¼ cup red wine vinegar

Directions

Preparing the Ingredients

1. In a large pot over medium-high heat, heat the olive oil until it shimmers.
2. Add the onions, celery, and carrots. Cook for 5 to 10 minutes, stirring occasionally, until the vegetables are soft.

Add the garlic and cook for 30 seconds, stirring constantly.

3. Stir in the lentils, bay leaves, broth, sea salt, pepper, and red pepper flakes. Bring to a simmer. Reduce the heat to medium-low and simmer for 10 minutes, stirring occasionally.

Remove and discard the bay leaves. Stir in the vinegar and serve.

Avgolemono (Lemon Chicken Soup)

Ingredients

½ large onion

2 medium carrots

1 celery stalk

1 garlic clove

5 cups low-sodium chicken stock

¼ cup brown rice

1½ cups (about 5 ounces) shredded rotisserie chicken

3 tablespoons freshly squeezed lemon juice

1 egg yolk

2 tablespoons chopped fresh dill

2 tablespoons chopped fresh parsley

Salt

Directions

Preparing the Ingredients

1. Place the onion, carrots, celery, and garlic in a food processor fitted with the chopping blade and pulse it until the vegetables are minced. You can also mince them by hand.

Add the vegetables and chicken stock to a stockpot or Dutch oven and bring it to a boil over high heat.

2. Reduce the heat to medium-low and add the rice, shredded chicken and lemon juice. Cover, and let the soup simmer for 40 minutes, or until the rice is cooked.

3. In a small bowl, whisk the egg yolk lightly. Very slowly, while whisking with one hand, pour about ½ of a ladle of the broth into the egg yolk to warm, or temper, the yolk. Slowly add another ladle of broth and continue to whisk.

Remove the soup from the heat and pour the whisked egg yolk–broth mixture into the pot. Stir well to combine.

Add the fresh dill and parsley. Season with salt, and serve.

Paella Soup

PREP TIME: 5 MINUTES / COOK TIME: 25 MINUTES/ SERVES 6

Ingredients

1 cup frozen green peas

2 tablespoons extra-virgin olive oil

1 cup chopped onion (about ½ medium onion)

1½ cups coarsely chopped red bell pepper (about 1 large pepper)

1½ cups coarsely chopped green bell pepper (about 1 large pepper)

2 garlic cloves, chopped (about 1 teaspoon)

1 teaspoon ground turmeric

1 teaspoon dried thyme

2 teaspoons smoked paprika

2½ cups uncooked instant brown rice

2 cups low-sodium or no-salt-added chicken broth

2½ cups water

1 (28-ounce) can low-sodium or no-salt-added crushed tomatoes

1 pound fresh raw medium shrimp (or frozen raw shrimp completely thawed), shells and tails removed

Directions

Preparing the Ingredients

1. Put the frozen peas on the counter to partially thaw as the soup is being prepared.
2. In a large stockpot over medium-high heat, heat the oil. Add the onion, red and green bell peppers, and garlic. Cook for 8 minutes, stirring occasionally. Add the turmeric, thyme, and smoked paprika, and cook for 2 minutes more, stirring often. Stir in the rice, broth, and water. Bring to a boil over high heat. Cover, reduce the heat to medium-low, and cook for 10 minutes.
3. Stir the peas, tomatoes, and shrimp into the soup. Cook for 4 to 6 minutes, until the shrimp is cooked, turning from gray to pink and white. The soup will be very thick, almost like stew, when ready to serve.

Roasted Eggplant Soup

PREP TIME: 15 MINUTES / COOK TIME: 40 MINUTES/ SERVES 6

Ingredients

2 pounds (1 to 2 medium to large) eggplant, halved lengthwise

2 beefsteak tomatoes, halved

2 onions, halved

4 garlic cloves, smashed

4 rosemary sprigs

2 tablespoons extra-virgin olive oil

1 to 2 cups no-salt-added vegetable stock

1 teaspoon pure maple syrup

1 teaspoon ground cumin

1 teaspoon ground coriander
1 teaspoon kosher salt
¼ teaspoon freshly ground black pepper
Lemon juice (optional)

Directions

Preparing the Ingredients

1. Preheat the oven to 400°F. Line two baking sheets with parchment paper or foil. Lightly spray with olive oil cooking spray. Spread the eggplant, tomatoes, onions, and garlic on the prepared baking sheets, cut-side down. Nestle the rosemary sprigs among the vegetables. Drizzle with the olive oil and roast for 40 minutes, checking halfway through and removing the garlic before it gets brown.

2. When cool enough to touch, remove the eggplant flesh and tomato flesh from the skin and add to a high-powered blender, food processor, or Vitamix.

3. Add the rosemary leaves, onions, garlic, 1 cup of the vegetable stock, maple syrup, cumin, coriander, salt, and black pepper. Purée until smooth.

4. The soup should be thick and creamy. If the soup is too thick, add another cup of stock slowly, until your desired consistency is reached. Spritz with lemon juice, if desired.

Chicken and Vegetable Soup

PREP TIME: 10 MINUTES / COOK TIME: 20 MINUTES/ SERVES 8

Ingredients

2 tablespoons extra-virgin olive oil

12 ounces boneless, skinless chicken breast, sliced

2 carrots, chopped

1 onion, chopped

1 red bell pepper, seeded and chopped

1 fennel bulb, chopped

5 garlic cloves, minced

6 cups unsalted chicken broth

1 (14-ounce) can crushed tomatoes, undrained

2 zucchini, chopped

1 tablespoon dried Italian seasoning

½ teaspoon sea salt

¼ teaspoon freshly ground black pepper

Directions

Preparing the Ingredients

1. In a large pot over medium-high heat, heat the olive oil until it shimmers.
2. Add the chicken and cook for about 5 minutes, stirring occasionally, until browned. Remove the chicken from the pot with a slotted spoon and set it aside.

Add the carrots, onion, red bell pepper, and fennel to the oil remaining in the pot. Cook for about 5 minutes, stirring occasionally, until the vegetables are soft.

Add the garlic and cook for 30 seconds, stirring constantly.

Stir in the broth, tomatoes, zucchini, Italian seasoning, sea salt, and pepper.

Bring to a boil, stirring occasionally. Reduce the heat and simmer for about 5 minutes more until the vegetables are soft.

Return the chicken to the pot. Cook for 1 minute more until the chicken heats through. Serve immediately.

To prepare the fennel bulb, cut off the stalks and reserve them for another use.

Cut the core from the bottom of the fennel in a "V" shape and discard. Halve the fennel lengthwise and chop. The remaining stalks can be added to salads, or cooked down like an onion to add to any dish.

Lentil Sweet Potato Soup

PREP TIME: 5 MINUTES / COOK TIME: 30 MINUTES/ SERVES 6

Ingredients

1 tablespoon extra-virgin olive oil

1 onion, diced

1 carrot, diced

1 celery stalk, diced

1 sweet potato, unpeeled and diced

1 cup green or brown lentils

1 dried bay leaf
1 teaspoon ground turmeric
1 teaspoon ground cumin
1 teaspoon kosher salt
¼ teaspoon freshly ground black pepper
4 cups no-salt-added vegetable stock

Directions

Preparing the Ingredients

Heat the olive oil in a large stockpot over medium-high heat. Add the onion, carrot, celery, and sweet potato and sauté 5 to 6 minutes. Add the lentils, bay leaf, turmeric, cumin, salt, and black pepper and cook for 30 seconds to 1 minute more.

Add the stock, bring to a boil, then lower the heat to low, and simmer, covered for 20 to 30 minutes, or until the lentils and sweet potato are tender. If you find the soup becoming thick and stew-like, feel free to add additional stock or water as it cooks. Herbs are a welcome addition to most dishes. If you have any fresh herbs, feel free to mix in ¼ cup chopped to the finished soup.

Zucchini and Meatball Soup

PREP TIME: 20 MINUTES / COOK TIME: 25 MINUTES/ SERVES 6

Ingredients

12 ounces ground turkey

1 yellow onion, grated and squeezed of excess water

1 tablespoon dried Italian seasoning

1 teaspoon garlic powder

1 teaspoon sea salt, divided

½ teaspoon freshly ground black pepper, divided

2 tablespoons extra-virgin olive oil

1 red onion, chopped

5 garlic cloves, minced

6 cups unsalted chicken broth

1 (14-ounce) can chopped tomatoes, drained

3 medium zucchini, chopped or spiralized

¼ cup chopped fresh basil leaves

Directions

Preparing the Ingredients

1. In a medium bowl, mix together the turkey, yellow onion, Italian seasoning, garlic powder, ½ teaspoon of sea salt, and ¼ teaspoon of pepper. On a plate, form the mixture into ¾-inch balls and set aside.

In a large pot over medium-high heat, heat the olive oil until it shimmers.

2. Add the red onion and cook for about 5 minutes, stirring occasionally, until soft. Add the garlic and cook for 30 seconds, stirring constantly.

Stir in the broth, tomatoes, remaining ½ teaspoon of salt, and remaining ¼ teaspoon of pepper. Bring to a boil. Add the meatballs and return to a boil. Reduce the heat to medium-low. Simmer for about 15 minutes, stirring occasionally, until the meatballs are cooked through.

Add the zucchini and cook for about 3 minutes more, until soft.

Stir in the basil just before serving.

Turmeric Red Lentil Soup

PREP TIME: 5 MINUTES / COOK TIME: 30 MINUTES/ SERVES 6

Ingredients

1 tablespoon extra-virgin olive oil

1 teaspoon ground cumin

1 teaspoon ground coriander

1 teaspoon ground turmeric

1 teaspoon kosher salt

¼ teaspoon freshly ground black pepper

1 tablespoon no-salt-added tomato paste

1 onion, diced

1 carrot, diced

1 celery stalk, diced
3 garlic cloves, minced
4 cups no-salt-added vegetable stock
2 cups water
1 cup red lentils
3 tablespoons lemon juice
¼ cup fresh parsley, chopped

Directions

Preparing the Ingredients

1. Heat the olive oil in a large stock pot over medium-high heat. Add the cumin, coriander, turmeric, salt, and black pepper and cook, stirring, for 30 seconds. Add the tomato paste and cook, stirring, for 30 seconds to 1 minute. Add the onion, carrot, and celery and sauté 5 to 6 minutes. Add the garlic and sauté 30 seconds.

2. Add the vegetable stock, water, and lentils and bring to a boil. Turn down the heat to low, and simmer, covering partially, until the lentils are tender, about 20 minutes. Mix in the lemon juice and parsley.

Tuscan Bean Soup with Kale

PREP TIME: 5 MINUTES / COOK TIME: 25 MINUTES/ SERVES 4

Ingredients

2 tablespoons extra-virgin olive oil

1 onion, diced

1 carrot, diced

1 celery stalk, diced

1 teaspoon kosher salt

4 cups no-salt-added vegetable stock

1 (15-ounce) can no-salt-added or low-sodium cannellini beans, drained and rinsed

1 tablespoon fresh thyme, chopped

1 tablespoon fresh sage, chopped

1 tablespoon fresh oregano, chopped

¼ teaspoon freshly ground black pepper

1 bunch kale, stemmed and chopped

¼ cup grated Parmesan cheese (optional)

Directions

Preparing the Ingredients

1. Heat the olive oil in a large pot over medium-high heat. Add the onion, carrot, celery, and salt and sauté until translucent and slightly golden, 5 to 6 minutes. Add the vegetable stock, beans, thyme, sage, oregano, and black pepper and bring to a boil. Turn down the heat to low, and simmer for 10 minutes. Stir in the kale and let it wilt, about 5 minutes. Sprinkle 1 tablespoon Parmesan cheese over each bowl before serving, if desired.

All-Purpose Chicken Broth (Instant Pot)

PREP TIME: 60 MINUTES / COOK TIME: 60 MINUTES/ SERVES 6 TO 8

Ingredients

3 pounds chicken wings

1 tablespoon vegetable oil

1 onion, chopped

3 garlic cloves, lightly crushed and peeled

12 cups water, divided

½ teaspoon table salt

3 bay leaves

Directions

1. Pat chicken wings dry with paper towels. Using highest sauté function, heat oil in Instant Pot for 5 minutes (or until just smoking). Brown half of chicken wings on all sides, about 10 minutes; transfer to bowl. Repeat with remaining chicken wings; transfer to bowl. Add onion to fat left in pot and cook until softened and well browned, 8 to 10 minutes. Stir in garlic and cook until fragrant, about 30 seconds. Stir in 1 cup water, scraping up any browned bits. Stir in remaining 11 cups water, salt, bay leaves, and chicken and any accumulated juices.

2. Lock lid in place and close pressure release valve. Select high pressure cook function and cook for 1 hour. Turn off Instant Pot and let pressure release naturally for 15 minutes. Quick-release any remaining pressure, then carefully remove lid, allowing steam to escape away from you.

3. Strain broth through fine-mesh strainer into large container, pressing on solids to extract as much liquid as possible; discard solids. Using wide, shallow spoon, skim excess fat from surface of broth. (Broth can be refrigerated for up to 4 days or frozen for up to 2 months.)

Moroccan-Style Chickpea Soup

PREP TIME: 5 MINUTES / COOK TIME: 30 MINUTES/ SERVES 4 TO 6

Ingredients

3 tablespoons extra-virgin olive oil

1 onion, chopped fine

1 teaspoon sugar

Salt and pepper

4 garlic cloves, minced

½ teaspoon hot paprika

¼ teaspoon saffron threads, crumbled

¼ teaspoon ground ginger

¼ teaspoon ground cumin

2 (15-ounce) cans chickpeas, rinsed

1 pound red potatoes, unpeeled, cut into ½-inch pieces

1 (14.5-ounce) can diced tomatoes

1 zucchini, cut into ½-inch pieces

3½ cups chicken or vegetable broth

¼ cup minced fresh parsley or mint

Lemon wedges

Directions

Preparing the Ingredients

1. Heat oil in Dutch oven over medium-high heat until shimmering. Add onion, sugar, and ½ teaspoon salt and cook until onion is softened, about 5 minutes. Stir in garlic, paprika, saffron, ginger, and cumin and cook until fragrant, about 30 seconds. Stir in chickpeas, potatoes, tomatoes and their juice, zucchini, and broth. Bring to simmer and cook, stirring occasionally, until potatoes are tender, 20 to 30 minutes.

2. Using wooden spoon, mash some of potatoes against side of pot to thicken soup. Off heat, stir in parsley and season with salt and pepper to taste. Serve with lemon wedges.

Vegetarian Mains
Socca Pan Pizza with Herbed Ricotta, Fresh Tomato, and Balsamic Glaze
PREP TIME: 15 MINUTES / COOK TIME: 15 MINUTES/ SERVES 2

Ingredients

1 cup chickpea flour

1 teaspoon baking powder

½ teaspoon salt

½ teaspoon garlic powder

½ teaspoon onion powder

1½ teaspoons Italian seasoning herb mix, divided

2 tablespoons grated Parmesan cheese

Up to 1 cup warm water

Olive oil, enough to coat the bottom of a skillet

½ cup ricotta cheese

1 ripe tomato, thinly sliced

Balsamic glaze

Directions

1. Preparing the Ingredients

Preheat the oven to 425°F and set the rack to the middle position.

While the oven is heating, combine the chickpea flour, baking powder, salt, garlic powder, onion powder, 1 teaspoon of the Italian seasoning herb mix, and the Parmesan cheese in a medium bowl.

Add most of the water and whisk to combine. The batter should be a pourable consistency like pancake batter, but not as thin as a crepe batter. You may not need all of the water.

2. Cooking.

Heat a large (10- to 12-inch) nonstick or cast iron skillet on the stovetop over medium-high heat and add the oil.

When the pan is hot, pour the batter into the pan and let it cook for a minute, until bubbles start to form. Transfer the pan to the oven and let it cook for 10 minutes, or until the batter starts to turn golden around the edges and looks set.

In a small bowl, combine the ricotta cheese and the remaining ½ teaspoon of Italian seasoning herb mix.

Remove the pan from the oven and gently spread the ricotta over the crust. Top with the sliced tomatoes and return to the oven for another 2 minutes to let the cheese melt.

Use a spatula to remove the dough from the pan. Drizzle it with balsamic glaze, slice, and serve.

Beet and Watercress Salad with Orange and Dill (Instant Pot)

Ingredients

2 pounds beets, scrubbed, trimmed, and cut into ¾-inch pieces
½ cup water
1 teaspoon caraway seeds
½ teaspoon table salt
1 cup plain Greek yogurt
1 small garlic clove, minced to paste
5 ounces (5 cups) watercress, torn into bite-size pieces
1 tablespoon extra-virgin olive oil, divided, plus extra for drizzling
1 tablespoon white wine vinegar, divided
1 teaspoon grated orange zest plus 2 tablespoons juice
¼ cup hazelnuts, toasted, skinned, and chopped
¼ cup coarsely chopped fresh dill
Coarse sea salt

Directions

Preparing the Ingredients

1. Combine beets, water, caraway seeds, and table salt in Instant Pot. Lock lid in place and close pressure release valve. Select high pressure cook function and cook for 8 minutes. Turn off Instant Pot and quick-release pressure. Carefully remove lid, allowing steam to escape away from you.

2. Using slotted spoon, transfer beets to plate; set aside to cool slightly. Combine yogurt, garlic, and 3 tablespoons beet cooking liquid in bowl; discard remaining cooking liquid. In large bowl toss watercress with 2 teaspoons oil and 1 teaspoon vinegar. Season with table salt and pepper to taste.

3. Spread yogurt mixture over surface of serving dish. Arrange watercress on top of yogurt mixture, leaving 1-inch border of yogurt mixture. Add beets to now-empty large bowl and toss with orange zest and juice, remaining 2 teaspoons vinegar, and remaining 1 teaspoon oil. Season with table salt and pepper to taste. Arrange beets on top of watercress mixture. Drizzle with extra oil and sprinkle with hazelnuts, dill, and sea salt.

Cauliflower Steaks with Olive Citrus Sauce

PREP TIME: 15 MINUTES / COOK TIME: 30 MINUTES / SERVES 4

Ingredients

1 or 2 large heads cauliflower (at least 2 pounds, enough for 4 portions)
⅓ cup extra-virgin olive oil
¼ teaspoon kosher salt
⅛ teaspoon ground black pepper
Juice of 1 orange
Zest of 1 orange
¼ cup black olives, pitted and chopped
1 tablespoon Dijon or grainy mustard

1 tablespoon red wine vinegar

½ teaspoon ground coriander

Directions

1. Preparing the Ingredients

Preheat the oven to 400°F. Line a baking sheet with parchment paper or foil.

Cut off the stem of the cauliflower so it will sit upright. Slice it vertically into four thick slabs. Place the cauliflower on the prepared baking sheet. Drizzle with the olive oil, salt, and black pepper.

2. **Cooking** . Bake for about 30 minutes, turning over once, until tender and golden brown.

In a medium bowl, combine the orange juice, orange zest, olives, mustard, vinegar, and coriander; mix well. Serve the cauliflower warm or at room temperature with the sauce.

Easy Brussels Sprouts Hash

PREP TIME: 5 MINUTES / COOK TIME: 20 MINUTES/ SERVES 4

Ingredients

3 tablespoons extra-virgin olive oil

1 onion, finely chopped

1 pound Brussels sprouts, bottoms trimmed off.

½ teaspoon caraway seeds

½ teaspoon sea salt

⅛ teaspoon freshly ground black pepper

¼ cup red wine vinegar

1 tablespoon Dijon mustard

1 tablespoon honey

3 garlic cloves, minced

Directions

Preparing the Ingredients

1. In a large skillet over medium-high heat, heat the olive oil until it shimmers. Add the onion, Brussels sprouts, caraway seeds, sea salt, and pepper. Cook for 7 to 10 minutes, stirring occasionally, until the Brussels sprouts begin to brown.

2. While the Brussels sprouts cook, whisk the vinegar, mustard, and honey in a small bowl and set aside.

Add the garlic to the skillet and cook for 30 seconds, stirring constantly.

Add the vinegar mixture to the skillet. Cook for about 5 minutes, stirring, until the liquid reduces by half.

An easy way to prepare the sprouts is to carefully grate them on a box grater, or use a mandoline set at ¼ inch with a guard. It allows you to have pieces of similar size so they cook evenly.

Caprese-Stuffed Portobellos

PREP TIME: 10 MINUTES / COOK TIME: 20 MINUTES/ SERVES 2

Ingredients

1 tablespoon olive oil, plus extra for drizzling

88

½ pint cherry or grape tomatoes

¼ teaspoon salt

Pinch freshly ground black pepper

3 medium garlic cloves, minced

4 to 5 large fresh basil leaves, thinly sliced, divided

2 large portobello mushrooms, stems removed

4 pieces mini mozzarella balls (ciliegine), halved

1 tablespoon grated Parmesan cheese

Directions

1. **Preparing the Ingredients. Preheat the oven to 350°F.**
2. **Cooking** . Heat 1 tablespoon of the olive oil in a sauté pan over medium-high heat. Add the tomatoes, salt, and pepper. Pierce a few of the tomatoes as they cook so they give off some juice. Cover and let the tomatoes soften for about 10 minutes. When the tomatoes are mostly softened and begin to break down, add the minced garlic and most of the basil—reserve about 2 teaspoons of basil to garnish at the end. Cook for 30 seconds and then remove from the heat.

Oil a baking pan and place the mushrooms gill-side up. If desired, season with salt and pepper. Divide the tomato mixture and the mozzarella balls between the mushrooms. Sprinkle the grated Parmesan cheese evenly over each and, if desired, drizzle the mushrooms with olive oil. Bake them for 20 minutes, or until the mushrooms are softened. If desired, place them under the broiler to brown the cheese a bit. Garnish with the remaining fresh basil.

Meze Plate with Hummus, Spiced Carrots, and Arugula(Instant Pot)

PREP TIME: 20 MINUTES / COOK TIME: 20 MINUTES/ MAKES ¼ CUP / SERVES 4

Ingredients

2 pounds carrots, peeled

½ cup chicken or vegetable broth

3 tablespoons Harissa (this page), divided

½ teaspoon table salt

2 ounces (2 cups) baby arugula

1 tablespoon extra-virgin olive oil

2 teaspoons lemon juice

1½ cups Hummus (this page)

½ cup Quick Pickled Onions (this page)

2 tablespoons roasted pepitas

Directions

Preparing the Ingredients

1. Cut carrots into 3-inch lengths. Leave thin pieces whole and halve larger pieces lengthwise. Combine carrots, broth, 1 tablespoon Harissa, and salt in Instant Pot. Lock lid in place and close pressure release valve. Select high pressure cook

function and cook for 1 minute. Turn off Instant Pot and quick-release pressure. Carefully remove lid, allowing steam to escape away from you; drain carrots.

2. Gently toss arugula with oil and lemon juice in bowl. Season with salt and pepper to taste. Spread portion of Hummus over bottom of individual serving plates. Using slotted spoon, arrange carrots on top and drizzle with remaining 2 tablespoons Harissa. Top with arugula, pickled onions, and pepitas.

Walnut Pesto Zoodles

PREP TIME: 15 MINUTES / COOK TIME: 10 MINUTES/ MAKES ¼ CUP / SERVES 4

Ingredients
4 medium zucchini (makes about 8 cups of zoodles)
¼ cup extra-virgin olive oil, divided
2 garlic cloves, minced (about 1 teaspoon), divided
½ teaspoon crushed red pepper
¼ teaspoon freshly ground black pepper, divided
¼ teaspoon kosher or sea salt, divided
2 tablespoons grated Parmesan cheese, divided
1 cup packed fresh basil leaves
¾ cup walnut pieces, divided

Directions
1. Preparing the Ingredients
Make the zucchini noodles (zoodles) using a spiralizer or your vegetable peeler to make ribbons (run the peeler down the zucchini to make long strips). In a large bowl, gently mix to combine the zoodles with 2 tablespoon of oil, 1 minced garlic clove, all the crushed red pepper, ⅛ teaspoon of black pepper, and ⅛ teaspoon of salt. Set aside.

2. Cooking
In a large skillet over medium-high heat, heat ½ tablespoon of oil. Add half of the zoodles to the pan and cook for 5 minutes, stirring every minute or so. Pour the cooked zoodles into a large serving bowl, and repeat with another ½ tablespoon of oil and the remaining zoodles. Add those zoodles to the serving bowl when they are done cooking. While the zoodles are cooking, make the pesto. If you're using a food processor, add the remaining minced garlic clove, ⅛ teaspoon of black pepper, and ⅛ teaspoon of salt, 1 tablespoon of Parmesan, all the basil leaves, and ¼ cup of walnuts. Turn on the processor, and slowly drizzle the remaining 2 tablespoons of oil into the opening until the pesto is completely blended. If you're using a high-powered blender, add the 2 tablespoons of oil first and then the rest of the pesto ingredients. Pulse until the pesto is completely blended. Add the pesto to the zoodles along with the remaining 1 tablespoon of Parmesan and the remaining ½ cup of walnuts. Mix together well and serve.

Pistachio Mint Pesto Pasta

PREP TIME: 10 MINUTES / COOK TIME: 10 MINUTES/ MAKES ¼ CUP / SERVES 4

Ingredients
8 ounces whole-wheat pasta
1 cup fresh mint

90

½ cup fresh basil

⅓ cup unsalted pistachios, shelled

1 garlic clove, peeled

½ teaspoon kosher salt

Juice of ½ lime

⅓ cup extra-virgin olive oil

Directions

Preparing the Ingredients

1. Cook the pasta according to the package directions. Drain, reserving ½ cup of the pasta water, and set aside.
2. In a food processor, add the mint, basil, pistachios, garlic, salt, and lime juice. Process until the pistachios are coarsely ground. Add the olive oil in a slow, steady stream and process until incorporated.
3. In a large bowl, mix the pasta with the pistachio pesto; toss well to incorporate. If a thinner, more saucy consistency is desired, add some of the reserved pasta water and toss well.

Roasted Asparagus with Lemon and Pine Nuts

PREP TIME: 5 MINUTES / COOK TIME: 20 MINUTES/ SERVES 4

Ingredients

1pound asparagus, trimmed

2 tablespoons extra-virgin olive oil

Juice of 1 lemon

Zest of 1 lemon

¼ cup pine nuts

½ teaspoon sea salt

⅛ teaspoon freshly ground black pepper

Directions

1. **Preparing the Ingredients**

Preheat the oven to 425°F.

In a large bowl, toss the asparagus with the olive oil, lemon juice and zest, pine nuts, sea salt, and pepper. Spread in a roasting pan in an even layer.

2. **Cooking**

Roast for about 20 minutes until the asparagus is browned.

Mushroom-Leek Tortilla de Patatas

PREP TIME: 30 MINUTES / COOK TIME:30 MINUTES, PLUS 5 MINUTES TO REST/ SERVES 2

Ingredients

1 tablespoon olive oil

1 cup thinly sliced leeks (from 1 leek, light green part only)

4 ounces baby bella (cremini) mushrooms, stemmed and sliced (about 1 cup)

1 small potato, peeled, sliced ¼-inch thick

5 large eggs, beaten

½ cup milk
1 teaspoon Dijon mustard
½ teaspoon dried thyme
½ teaspoon salt
Pinch freshly ground black pepper
3 ounces Gruyère cheese, shredded

Directions

Preparing the Ingredients

1. Preheat the oven to 350°F and set the rack to the middle position.

Heat the olive oil in a large sauté pan (nonstick is best) over medium-high heat. Add the leeks, mushrooms, and potato slices and sauté until the leeks are golden and the potatoes start to brown, about 10 minutes.

2. Reduce the heat to medium-low, cover the pan, and let the vegetables cook for another 10 minutes, or until the potatoes begin to soften. If the potato slices stick to the bottom of the pan, add 1 to 2 tablespoons of water to the pan, but be careful because it may splatter.

3. While the vegetables are cooking, combine the beaten eggs, milk, mustard, thyme, salt, pepper, and cheese in a medium bowl and whisk everything together.

4. When the potatoes are soft enough to pierce with a fork or knife, turn off the heat.

Transfer the cooked vegetables to an oiled 8-inch oven-safe pan (nonstick is best) and arrange them in a nice layer along the bottom and slightly up the sides of the pan. Alternatively, you can use a glass pie or quiche dish. A smaller pan will give you a nice, tall, moist omelet.

5. Pour the egg mixture over the vegetables and give it a light shake or tap to distribute the eggs evenly through the vegetables.

Bake the tortilla for 25 to 30 minutes, or until the eggs are set and the top is golden and puffed. Remove it from the oven, and let it sit for 5 minutes before cutting into it.

Rustic Garlic Toasts with Stewed Tomatoes, Shaved Fennel, and Burrata (Instnt Pot)

Ingredients

2 tablespoons extra-virgin olive oil, divided, plus extra for drizzling
5 garlic cloves, sliced thin
1½ teaspoons fennel seeds, lightly cracked
1 (28-ounce) can whole peeled tomatoes, drained with juice reserved, halved
⅛ teaspoon table salt
8 ounces burrata cheese, room temperature
1 fennel bulb, stalks discarded, bulb halved, cored, and sliced thin
4 ounces (4 cups) baby arugula
1 recipe Garlic Toasts (this page)
Balsamic glaze
Coarse sea salt

Directions

Preparing the Ingredients

1. Using highest sauté function, cook 1 tablespoon oil, garlic, and fennel seeds in Instant Pot until fragrant and garlic is light-golden brown, about 3 minutes. Stir in tomatoes and reserved juice and table salt. Lock lid in place and close pressure release valve. Select high pressure cook function and cook for 2 minutes.

2. Turn off Instant Pot and quick-release pressure. Carefully remove lid, allowing steam to escape away from you. Continue to cook tomato mixture using highest sauté function until sauce is slightly thickened, about 5 minutes.

3. Place burrata on plate and cut into rough 1½-inch pieces, collecting creamy liquid. Toss fennel and arugula with remaining 1 tablespoon oil in large bowl. Season with table salt and pepper to taste. Arrange toasts on individual serving plates and top with tomato mixture, fennel-arugula salad, and burrata and any accumulated liquid. Drizzle with glaze and extra oil, and sprinkle with sea salt.

Cauliflower Steaks with Eggplant Relish

Ingredients

2 small heads cauliflower (about 3 pounds)
¼ teaspoon kosher or sea salt
¼ teaspoon smoked paprika
Extra-virgin olive oil, divided

Directions

1. **Preparing the Ingredients**

Place a large, rimmed baking sheet in the oven. Preheat the oven to 400°F with the pan inside. Stand one head of cauliflower on a cutting board, stem-end down. With a long chef's knife, slice down through the very center of the head, including the stem. Starting at the cut edge, measure about 1 inch and cut one thick slice from each cauliflower half, including as much of the stem as possible, to make two cauliflower "steaks." Reserve the remaining cauliflower for another use. Repeat with the second cauliflower head.

Dry each steak well with a clean towel. Sprinkle the salt and smoked paprika evenly over both sides of each cauliflower steak.

2. **Cooking**

In a large skillet over medium-high heat, heat 2 tablespoons of oil. When the oil is very hot, add two cauliflower steaks to the pan and cook for about 3 minutes, until golden and crispy. Flip and cook for 2 more minutes. Transfer the steaks to a plate. Use a pair of tongs to hold a paper towel and wipe out the pan to remove most of the hot oil (which will contain a few burnt bits of cauliflower). Repeat the cooking process with the remaining 2 tablespoons of oil and the remaining two steaks.

Using oven mitts, carefully remove the baking sheet from the oven and place the cauliflower on the baking sheet. Roast in the oven for 12 to 15 minutes, until the cauliflower steaks are just fork tender; they will still be somewhat firm. Serve the steaks with the Eggplant Relish Spread, baba ghanoush, or the homemade ketchup from our Italian Baked Beans recipe.

Burst Cherry Tomato Sauce with Angel Hair Pasta

PREP TIME: 10 MINUTES / COOK TIME: 20 MINUTES/ SERVES 4

Ingredients

8 ounces angel hair pasta

2 tablespoons extra-virgin olive oil

3 garlic cloves, minced

3 pints cherry tomatoes

½ teaspoon kosher salt

¼ teaspoon red pepper flakes

¾ cup fresh basil, chopped

1 tablespoon white balsamic vinegar (optional)

¼ cup grated Parmesan cheese (optional)

Directions

1. Cook the pasta according to the package directions. Drain and set aside.
2. Heat the olive oil in a skillet or large sauté pan over medium-high heat. Add the garlic and sauté for 30 seconds. Add the tomatoes, salt, and red pepper flakes and cook, stirring occasionally, until the tomatoes burst, about 15 minutes.
3. Remove from the heat and add the pasta and basil. Toss together well. (For out-of-season tomatoes, add the vinegar, if desired, and mix well.)

Serve with the grated Parmesan cheese, if desired.

Citrus Sautéed Spinach

PREP TIME: 5 MINUTES / COOK TIME: 5 MINUTES/ SERVES 4

Ingredients

2 tablespoons extra-virgin olive oil

4 cups fresh baby spinach

1 teaspoon orange zest

¼ cup freshly squeezed orange juice

½ teaspoon sea salt

⅛ teaspoon freshly ground black pepper

Directions

1. Preparing the Ingredients

In a large skillet over medium-high heat, heat the olive oil until it shimmers. Add the spinach and orange zest. Cook for about 3 minutes, stirring occasionally, until the spinach wilts. Stir in the orange juice, sea salt, and pepper. Cook for 2 minutes more, stirring occasionally. Serve hot. Before serving, add ¼ cup chopped walnuts for crunch. The recipe also works with kale or Swiss chard, but increase the cooking time to about 10 minutes.

Gnocchi with Creamy Butternut Squash and Blue Cheese Sauce

PREP TIME: 10 MINUTES / COOK TIME: 20 MINUTES/ SERVES 2

Ingredients

5 ounces frozen diced butternut squash
¼ cup low-sodium vegetable stock
Pinch salt
Pinch nutmeg
Pinch cayenne pepper
Pinch freshly ground black pepper
8 ounces prepared, packaged gnocchi
1 tablespoon olive oil
1 garlic clove, minced
2 fresh sage leaves
1 ounce Gorgonzola Dolce or other mild blue cheese
1 tablespoon heavy cream (optional)

Directions

1. Preparing the Ingredients

In a saucepan, bring the butternut squash and vegetable stock to a boil. Cover, and reduce the heat to medium-low. Simmer for 10 minutes, or until the squash is very tender.

Transfer the squash and vegetable stock to a blender. Add the salt, nutmeg, cayenne, and black pepper, and blend on low speed until it's completely smooth. (Make sure your blender is no more than half full or the hot liquid may erupt through the lid.) Taste and add additional salt if needed. Set the squash aside.

Using the same saucepan, cook the gnocchi according to package directions. While the gnocchi cooks, heat the olive oil in a large sauté pan over medium-high heat. Add the garlic and sage and sauté for 45 seconds, just until the garlic and sage are fragrant. Carefully add the puréed squash to the sauté pan. Stir in the cheese and cream, if using. Add the cooked gnocchi to the pan and gently stir to coat with the sauce. Taste and add any salt, pepper, or another pinch of nutmeg as needed. Remove the sage leaves before serving. Gnocchi are made from potato and flour and they cook very quickly. Make sure you remove them from the heat as soon as the gnocchi float to the top of the pan. I like to use a slotted spoon and scoop them right from the water and into the sauce.

Mediterranean Lentil Sloppy Joes

PREP TIME: 5 MINUTES / COOK TIME: 15 MINUTES/ SERVES 4

Ingredients

1 tablespoon extra-virgin olive oil

1 cup chopped onion (about ½ medium onion)

1 cup chopped bell pepper, any color (about 1 medium bell pepper)

2 garlic cloves, minced (about 1 teaspoon)

1 (15-ounce) can lentils, drained and rinsed

1 (14.5-ounce) can low-sodium or no-salt-added diced tomatoes, undrained

1 teaspoon ground cumin

1 teaspoon dried thyme

¼ teaspoon kosher or sea salt

4 whole-wheat pita breads, split open

1½ cups chopped seedless cucumber (1 medium cucumber)

1 cup chopped romaine lettuce

Directions

Preparing the Ingredients

1. In a medium saucepan over medium-high heat, heat the oil. Add the onion and bell pepper and cook for 4 minutes, stirring frequently. Add the garlic and cook for 1 minute, stirring frequently. Add the lentils, tomatoes (with their liquid), cumin, thyme, and salt. Turn the heat to medium and cook, stirring occasionally, for 10 minutes, or until most of the liquid has evaporated.

2. Stuff the lentil mixture inside each pita. Lay the cucumbers and lettuce on top of the lentil mixture and serve.